Heal Hashimoto's:
Start with the Gut

Dr. Sharon Lee Rasa

Disclaimer:

The medical information in this book is provided as an educational resource only, and is not intended to be used or relied upon for any diagnostic or treatment purposes. This information should not be used as a substitute for professional diagnosis and treatment

The lifestyle interventions discussed in this book should not be used as a substitute for conventional medical therapy.

Furthermore, none of the statements in this book have been evaluated by the Food and Drug Administration.

Please consult your healthcare provider before making any health care decisions or for guidance about a specific medical condition

ISBN-10: 1533360006
ISBN-13: 978-1533360007

Dedication: To all the patients who have allowed me the privilege to serve them on their journey to health and healing.

Contents

Acknowledgements 1

1. My Aha Moment 3

2. Doc... Could It Be My Thyroid? 7

3. Diagnosis and Testing 15

4. Your Living Gut 27

5. Sick to my gut 37

6. It's a Gut Feeling 49

7. The Nourished Gut 55

8. 5 R's: Remove, Replenish, Repair, Re-inoculate, Rebalance 67

9. Gut Solutions 87

10. Gut Bless You 111

Resources 117

About the Author 121

Acknowledgements

First I am grateful to my Father in Heaven through whom all things are possible. I am grateful to my own body for providing me not only a place to live, but also for being a living laboratory that I could experiment on and learn from.

To my husband, Tom, who always has my back and encourages me, loves me, and believes in me in a way I have never known.

To my son, Jason, and daughter-in-law, Amy Lee, for providing us with five endearing grandchildren who inspire me to live well, work hard, and love more.

To the founders of the Hashimoto's Institute: Dr. Izabella Wentz, Dr. Christianson, and Andrea Nakayama for leading the way in helping millions find their root cause in Hashimoto's Autoimmune Disease.

To Dietrich Klinghardt, MD, Ph.d, the *people's* doctor.

My Aha Moment

Heal Hashimoto's – Start with the Gut!

At nearly 60 years young I was pleased I was able to participate in a yearly Jersey Girl Triathlon: Ocean swim 300yds, 11-mile bike ride, and 3-mile walk/run. It was not an Iron Man by any definition, but it certainly required a level of fitness and ability I was grateful to have.

I was not on any medications but my health history did include Lyme disease and mold exposure.

Having been in the natural health field for most of my adult life I treated my body mostly through herbals, homeopathic medicine, and alternative holistic therapies. I was grateful to remain symptom free as long as I kept a moderate level of ongoing self-care to keep my body optimized and fueled.

I only go to the medical doctor one time a year, and that is to have a physical and routine blood work done. This year was different, as I sat in her office and explained that I felt more tired than I had in years. I said my skin and hair were very dry and I had gained 10 pounds in a relatively short period of time, even though my diet had not changed significantly. Her reply was, "It was an awful winter... everybody gained weight." I then said, "Doc, could it be my thyroid?" She said she would include some thyroid panels in the blood work and I left.

A week later her office called to say that my thyroid came back positive and she wanted me to go on medicine right away. These were unfamiliar words for me. I was not on medicine and I was not eager to start. I am not against pharmaceutics, but as a natural health practitioner I had seen a long history of patients on way too many meds, often causing the very symptoms they were prescribed for. I asked to make an appointment to see the doctor to discuss her recommendations.

That visit left me a bit stunned. The doctor said I would need to be on thyroid medication for the rest of my life. When I asked, "Why?" she impatiently said, "Because your thyroid is NOT working!" My reply was, "And I don't think this medicine is going to make it work."

Her first recommendation was synthroid, and I asked her about some alternatives, such as Nature Throid and Westhroid. She said if I wanted to she would give me a prescription for that. I told her I needed some time to think about it and I would get back to her. Over the next few weeks I thought long and hard about my visit with her, and the fact that she never asked me about anything in my life that may have contributed to this extreme change in TSH levels from one year to the next.

I began to think back over the previous few months in my life, and I soon realized a lot of things had happened.

For one, I had a younger brother who had become quite ill. Severely ill, in fact, and we were afraid we would lose him. I had invited him to come and live with me and my husband so that I could provide him with a natural approach that would involve major lifestyle changes. So he moved in with us and I took total responsibility for his health care, including taking him to my office every day and working on him between my other patients. He slept a lot of the time. I cooked for him and massaged him and cared for him and prayed over him. I desperately did not want him to die and I was an emotional wreck.

During that time my own self-care suffered, and I was not as vigilant about my meditation, exercise, and other healthy practices. I also became gluten free, but I made a huge mistake when I replaced gluten with many of the gluten-free processed foods that are available on the market. Many gluten-free foods are made by replacing wheat flour with cornstarch, rice starch, potato starch, or tapioca starch. While they do not trigger the immune or neurological response of wheat gluten, they do trigger the glucose-insulin response that causes you to gain weight. Wheat products increase blood sugar and insulin more than most other foods. But foods made with cornstarch, rice starch, potato starch and tapioca starch are among the few foods that increase blood sugar even MORE than wheat products. Gluten-free foods come with a lot of consequences.

This combined with the emotional stress of potentially losing my brother and best friend as well as running a busy natural care practice was overwhelming for me.

I became a little angry that this doctor's only solution was for me to go on medication for the rest of my life. As a chiropractor and now a trained functional medicine practitioner, this suggestion that I would never be healed or cured but the medicine would help with symptoms left me questioning the entire process.

My personal and professional philosophy is that the body has an innate intelligence that directs every cellular function. I had personally witnessed hundreds of patients in my care who were given poor diagnoses of everything from diabetes to cancer and RA to fibromyalgia, who not only recovered but were cured... so why not me?

Heal Hashimoto's: Start with the Gut is based not only on my personal journey, but my professional one as well. Good food is not the same as the "right" food. Some of my sickest patients have improved the most by addressing the right food for them. Remember, food sensitivity is not the same as food allergy. How do we know the difference? This is part of what we will address in *Heal Hashimoto's*. Going gluten, dairy, or sugar free can be an overwhelming challenge for many people. "What do I eat?" is the first question. "Where do I find the time?" "How do I implement these changes?" We will also address these in *Heal Hashimoto's*.

As a graduate of the Hashimoto's Institute and through hundreds of post-graduate hours in Functional Medicine, I was trained and aptly able to help hundreds of others navigate this often hazy and misdirected path. Now I hope I can be of help to you too!

Doc... Could It Be My Thyroid?

You just don't have the kind of energy you used to... You wake up in the morning and want to hide under the covers... In this chapter you'll begin to see if you relate to any of the symptoms of Hashimoto's. People with Hashimoto's pronounced (hash-e-moat-ohs) may have a few things in common and differ on many others. We'll learn the three things all Hashimoto's patients have in common.

Possible Symptoms

- Drier and/or itchy skin
- Constipation
- Numbness & tingling
- Premature balding and diffuse hair loss
- Weight Gain
- Drier, coarser, more brittle hair
- Fatigue & tendency to fall asleep during the day
- Your tongue may be abnormally large and the sides may be scalloped
- Low basal temperature
- Red, irritated, dry eyes
- Night vision problems are frequent
- Hoarseness
- Paresthesias, tingling, burning sensation
- Dizziness and vertigo
- Sleep apnea
- Depression
- Vertigo or tinnitus
- Mild elevation of liver enzymes

- Elevated cholesterol
- Infertility
- Headaches & migraines
- Fibromyalgia
- Water retention
- Voice change or hoarseness
- Puffy eyes
- Palpitations
- Shortness of breath
- Vitiligo
- Low Vitamin D Levels
- Low ferritin, low iron (anemia)
- Kidney stones, infection
- Joint pain and stiffness
- Insulin resistance
- Adrenal fatigue
- GERD (gastroesophageal reflux disease)
- Eczema
- Chronic Candida
- Cold all the time
- Nutrient deficiency, despite good diet
- Thinning eyebrows
- Throat discomfort, swelling or frequent sore throats
- Irritability

Do you know that Thyroid disease is the most under-diagnosed disorder and the most mistreated condition?

Sadly, most Doc's really miss the mark here. When a thyroid disorder is identified, the standard of care since the 1960's is the prescribed medication of T4, which can be found under brand names such as: Synthroid or Levoxyl. Doctors are taught the problem is just in the thyroid, when most of the time it is not. T4 is a storage hormone. Your thyroid also produces T3, T2, T1 and calcitonin. For many, taking T4 is like taking an elevator that only goes to the 5th floor when you are trying to get to the penthouse.

Most doctors simply address the thyroid without considering the underlying issue. You could be one of the estimated **80% of**

people who have an autoimmune thyroid condition, meaning that you body is confused as to which proteins are foreign and invaders and which are helpful and necessary. Our immune system is designed to recognize, attack, and destroy invaders. This can be a real problem if the body confuses the friend for the foe.

All dis-ease is our body messaging us that something needs to change… and that change does not happen in a pill.

Unfortunately, many people are being treated for thyroid conditions with replacement hormones, and yet still suffering with a multitude of unexplainable symptoms. This can be true for so many because the doctor points to their "normal" blood work, and therefore the "success" of the medication. **Of course there is a time and a place for medication, especially if you are one of those who do not have a thyroid.**

What does the thyroid do?

I'm glad you asked. When it's working properly we sort of take it for granted that we have plenty of energy, our bodies feel cold and warm when they are supposed to, we maintain the right weight, and our mood is stable and reliable.

All of these controls are influenced by the proper functioning of our thyroid gland.

Thyroid Anatomy

Imagine wearing a bowtie. The area that it would cover is where you would find the thyroid. It sits just below your larynx. The thyroid gland is shaped like a butterfly and is about the size of a deck of cards when it is normal.

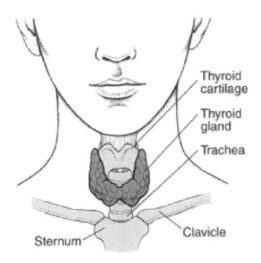

The thyroid is comprised of hundreds of tiny follicles, and each of those follicles is creating thyroid hormone. The thyroid needs a lot of iodine to work, so there is a special pump that pulls iodine from the bloodstream into the thyroid. This pump pulls iodine inside the thyroid and binds it to something called thyroglobulin. The thyroid gland does a big job by combining two rather simple substances, which together make thyroid hormone. One of these is iodine. The other is Thyroxine, a common amino acid found in most proteins. These amino acids are either manufactured easily in the body or obtained from the digestion of protein in the diet.

The problem is not necessarily a lack of the ingredients, but more a disruption in the assembly phase. Normally, these building blocks undergo a series of reactions resulting in the attachment of four atoms of iodine to one molecule of tyrosine. This product is called T-4. It is one of the two main thyroid hormones and the one most commonly measured. It is also called the least bioactive because in its circulating form it cannot bind to the cell nucleus material.

T-3 is what we get when T-4 gives up one atom of iodine. Its full name is triiodothyronine and it is the active hormone. Thyroglobulin is taken with the iodine inside the follicle, and those undergo chemical reactions that make up the T numbers. T3, T4, etc.

T3 means there are 3 iodines attached, and T4 means there are 4 iodines. When we are stacking on iodine we are forming thyroid hormones, and when we are using hormones it is the exact opposite. Once the hormones leave the thyroid, by pulling off iodine atoms we go from T4 to T3 to T2 to T1, and we call it deiodination (removing iodine).

About 20 percent of T4 is converted to T3 in the GI tract and about 80% happens in the liver.

How does this all happen? Certain enzymes are responsible for taking T4 and converting it to active T3 or inactive (reverse T3). The body actually makes more reverse T3 than active T3, and the reason is the body makes more thyroid hormone than it thinks it needs because it never wants to run out of it. Most of the thyroid hormone we make we get rid of by a process of converting it into reverse T3. T3 is is further broken down into T2. We don't hear much about T2, but it is a metabolically active hormone.

This regulation begins when the hypothalamus sends messages to the pituitary by putting out TRH, or Thyroid Releasing Hormone. TRH stimulates the pituitary to make TSH, or Thyroid Stimulating Hormone. The hypothalamus is like the CEO and the pituitary is the regional manager. The pituitary is dealing directly with the thyroid, the adrenals, the testicles, the ovaries, and more.

The thyroid is part of the most complicated system in your entire body. You need to run the correct panel of numbers to get a more precise understanding of the clinical picture. This is a big bone of contention in many medical offices because the Standard of Care dictates they only evaluate the TSH level (Thyroid Stimulating Hormone), and maybe T3 and T4. There is a great deal of controversy around this approach, as conventional doctors have adopted TSH as the "Gold Standard." If the TSH is normal, the search for hypothyroidism usually ends.

The problem here is many people with thyroid disease have normal TSH levels because TSH is a Pituitary hormone. Unfortunately, this test cannot measure if all your cells and tissues are receiving the released thyroid hormones. If you are, the TSH result will be normal. The best way to use the TSH lab test is in diagnosing a pituitary problem, not a thyroid problem.

A very low TSH with a low free T3 gives away a pituitary issue. As a certified practitioner of Dr. Klinghardt's work, I often hear him in the back of my mind saying, "Treat the patient... not the lab!"

Patients often go undiagnosed or misdiagnosed because the standard of care for testing is to only test for TSH, Thyroid Stimulating Hormone. If it falls in the so-called "normal range," the doc says you're fine and sends you on your way.

Thyroid hormone influences the way that cholesterol and other lipids are synthesized and broken down, and this happens in the liver. This is one of the reasons people with Hashimoto's and hypothyroidism often have lipid panels with imbalances in their cholesterol, LDL, and triglycerides.

So what could go wrong?

The big picture is in the genes. One group of HLA genes causes the thyroid to become goitrous or thickened, or enlarged or nodular. Another variant of those HLA genes causes the gland to get broken down. They both cause structural changes and they're both part of Hashimoto's process, which is why a diagnostic ultrasound can be so beneficial. It's important to know just because you have the gene does not mean your future is predetermined. Current research focuses on the "epigenetics" which will affect whether or not that gene is expressed.

Because this is an X-linked trait it is more common among women. If you are genetically prone, it does not take a great deal of environmental stressors to trigger it.

Another thing that can go wrong is immune dysregulation, and many things can trigger that, including low Vitamin D and infections.

Three factors must be present in order for Hashimoto's to occur

#1 Genetic Predisposition

#2 Leaky Gut/Intestinal permeability

#3 Microbial Make-up/infection

All dis-ease is our body messaging us that something needs to change... and that change does not happen in a pill.

What's the bottom line?

Take Action!

Become informed. You must be your own advocate. After reading this book you will likely be more informed than many doctors.

Find a practitioner who will run the correct labs and is able to interpret them. Then differentiate the treatment accordingly.

Chapter summary

- ✓ Symptoms may vary
- ✓ Healing does not happen in a pill
- ✓ Be your own advocate
- ✓ Run the correct labs and have them interpreted by a skilled practitioner
- ✓ What Hashimoto patients have in common: Genetic predisposition, leaky gut, and infection.

Diagnosis and Testing

When I first went into practice, I was told to sign on with every insurance provider that you could. One of the reasons is because you, the patient, will log onto their insurance provider account and then "choose" a doc that is IN network, and I, as a provider, would receive many referrals from the network. That made sense at the time.

Once I was "IN" network I found the catch. You see… if it sounds too good to be true… it probably is. Insurance providers I had contracted with would tell me what I could do for a patient, when I could do it for a patient, and how many times I could do it for a patient… Not to mention how much I should be paid. What's the problem with that? Insurance companies are corporations with shareholders and their objective is to MAKE money. That's the bottom line. I, on the other hand, have an objective to provide the best care possible for my patients. We are in direct conflict with our objectives. Insurance companies want to offer patients the least amount of tools, therapies, treatments for the shortest amount of time in order to build revenue for their shareholders. Their "Standard of care" is based on a "sick care" model and not a "wellness" model. Let me give you some examples:

When you go for a yearly physical, the insurance company already has a list of the "approved" tests needed for "standard of care." The unfortunate part is that this list does not PAY for many of the most important biomarkers that Functional Medicine and Integrative practitioners rely on to understand inflammation, infection, or things like predisposing factors. Even Vitamin D, which is essential, is often an "add on" to the list, and patients have to pay a lot of money to get the testing that is needed which exceeds the approved list.

Years ago I had frozen shoulder. As a Chiropractor this can be a BIG deal, as I am unable to perform the actions to do my work. Nothing I tried, including standard physical therapy, was resolving the condition 100%. I learned about a device that I could use at home to traction my shoulder on a daily basis with no side effects, user friendly, and 80% effective. I wanted one!

The device was available for rent at $480/month. When I contacted my insurance company to cover the cost they asked me if I had had the approved surgery for frozen shoulder. I replied, "No, that is why I need the traction device, because I want to avoid surgery." Their reply was if I had the surgery and it was unsuccessful they would cover the cost of the traction device. I was astounded. You mean to tell me you would rather pay thousands of dollars for a surgery I may not need than $480 a month? The reply, "That is our standard of care!" For me, I decided to pay out of pocket and get the device, which did resolve the shoulder 100%!

I began to think of all the family members and patients who told me about procedures, surgeries, and other invasive treatments they selected because that is WHAT INSURANCE WOULD PAY FOR! The big takeaway here is your insurance company is not looking out for what is best for you; they are looking for what is best for their shareholders!

Think about it... every time you call a doctor's office, before they even ask you your name, they ask you, "What insurance do you have?" The reason being: before the doctor ever sees you face to face they already know what tests they can and cannot run and will determine your care based on how they will or won't be paid. This is simply wrong.

Now more and more alternative practitioners are going to a cash model. I am one of them. When a patient walks through my door, they are paying me their hard-earned dollars, and I feel a responsibility to deliver the best care possible. Often that care is very, very different than what their insurance company deems standard.

Like many of you, I have insurance. It costs a lot of money and I rarely use it. Why? The doctors I want to use have a cash practice and my deductible for out-of-network is $10,000! Therefore, I do what many of my patients do, and that is pay for everything out of pocket. I can't afford to be sick and neither can you. We cannot afford to not work, not care for our families, and not be able to meet our financial obligations.

This is only one of the reasons I am writing this book. We can get well. We must learn how and what we need to do that. Our bodies are self-healing, self-regulating organisms, and given no interference they have the innate wisdom to deliver the right medicine at the right time in the proper dosage.

Having explained this insurance model, perhaps now you can understand that the standard tests to determine if you have a thyroid condition are limited to TSH and T4. This is not because these are the best tests, but these are the approved standard of care your doctor and your insurance company will most likely pay for. Sadly, this leaves millions of people walking around underdiagnosed, misdiagnosed, and over- and under-treated.

According to the American Association of Clinical Endocrinologists, more than 27 million Americans suffer from thyroid dysfunction, half of whom go undiagnosed by conventional medicine. Of the detected cases of hypothyroidism, 90 percent are due to Hashimoto's disease. Thyroid replacement hormones ignore what caused the thyroid to become depressed in the first place. For example, irregular immune function, poor blood sugar metabolism, gut infections, adrenal problems, and hormonal imbalance can all significantly depress thyroid function.

Diagnostic ultrasound is one of the most useful and informative tests for someone with a thyroid condition. Typically, if you do not ask the doc to perform one, they will never mention it to you. Epstein-Barr virus is one of the most likely infections we find in a thyroid patient, and most docs not only do not run the test, but they never link it to a possible thyroid condition. So, what happens next? These patients end up in practitioner's offices like mine with growing nodules, enlarged or atrophic thyroid glands, depressed and in despair with what they call a MYSTERY ILLNESS. IT IS ONLY A MYSTERY ILLNESS IF YOU DO NOT KNOW WHAT TO LOOK FOR!!!

Derived from the Greek word meaning "shield," the thyroid is a butterfly-shaped gland that sits right below the Adam's apple. Its main job is to regulate metabolism – the ability to break down food and convert it to energy. I like to think of the thyroid as the "sun" in our body. Like the sun, it is providing us with the life-giving essence for the body to do its work. When the thyroid is imbalanced, patients report that the "zest" has gone out of life. They feel tired and lifeless. So you can see keeping the thyroid functioning is essential to the quality of life.

What happens in Hashimoto's is a combination called the "perfect storm." Genetic predisposition with leaky gut, and the added fire of infections. Hashimoto's Thyroiditis is an autoimmune condition that may result in destruction of the thyroid gland. Hashimoto's is the most common cause of hypothyroidism in the United States, and accounts for 90% of cases of hypothyroidism. This condition was first described by Hakuro Hashimoto, a Japanese physician.

So let's talk about the tests that are important when considering a thyroid condition.

Basic Tests:

- TSH
- TPO Antibodies
- Thyroglobulin Antibodies
- Free T4
- Free T3
- Reverse T3

Typically, Hashimoto's disorder will reveal one or two types of anti-thyroid antibodies. Thyroid peroxidase (TPO) antibody is the most common, followed by Thyroglobulin Antibodies.

Today, there is emerging research to suggest that Thyroid Releasing Hormone can be helpful in identifying thyroid disorders earlier than TSH. It turns out there was a time when all doctors used the TRH, but as medicine advances and assays became more sensitive, the TSH replaced TRH and is now the accepted way to diagnose.thyroid disorders. Once again, due to rising costs and saving money, the system moved to an easier and less expensive draw by only testing for TSH.

Because there are stages of Hashimoto's, these lab numbers can vary from test to test and it takes a trained eye to interpret what the numbers are revealing.

In our office we begin with a thorough history. We have every patient fill out a 16-page questionnaire, and we ask everything from their birth history to their dental history, and their emotional trauma to their life's work.

We follow this up with Heart Rate Variability[1] scanning and Autonomic Response Testing[2]. Heart rate variability is an in-office screening that provides us with information on how well the Autonomic Nervous System is functioning. Many patients have a revved-up sympathetic nervous system and are not getting the repair and rest they need at night when the parasympathetic nervous system is most active. This simple scan guides our treatment and is an invaluable tool to monitor patients' progress.

Autonomic Response Testing was developed as an offshoot of Applied Kinesiology. It is a more refined muscle testing, and in the hands of a skilled practitioner, the information we can glean from the body provides a roadmap in both understanding the root cause and what treatment(s) will be most efficacious for the patient we are working with.

No two patients with the same diagnosis respond to the same treatment. Practitioners who embrace "muscle testing," have come to find the results to be more reliable than most of the lab work

---

[1] http://rasahealth.com/2011/09/heart-rate-variability-a-useful-tool/
[2] http://rasahealth.com/what-is-autonomic-response-testing/

they may have used. Over the years, patients who have come to us have seen a considerable number of highly qualified practitioners and still are not satisfied with their results. Being skilled in Autonomic Response Testing gives the practitioner an edge in uncovering root issues that may have gone undetected in traditional lab testing, and can then be treated accordingly.

Blood, urine, hair, and stool testing are also part of our doctor's black bag. They are valuable tools, but there are many false positives and false negatives. Often split samples sent to the same lab can come back with different results. Before I suggest medication or treatment for my patients, I want to build a case that leaves little room for doubt and not make a life-long decision based on one biomarker that may be incorrect or misleading.

When choosing a practitioner, be mindful of their background and training. Every practitioner, including myself, has a bias toward their speciality and their philosophical model. If you asked a conventionally-trained endocrinologist which is the best thyroid medication, you will typically hear Synthroid. If you ask how long you will have to take it, their reply is often, "The rest of your life."

If you ask someone trained in Functional and Integrative Medicine, they will often ask, "What is the root cause of your thyroid disorder?" Every thyroid disorder I know of is impacted by the gut. No matter what your mystery illness or thyroid autoimmune diagnosis may or may not be, I promise you you will benefit by not only understanding the role of the gut but learning how to heal it.

There is a lot to know about testing and diagnosis for Hashimoto's. The author assumes most people reading this book will have already been diagnosed or considering a differential diagnosis. Therefore, do not rely on this information for this important and necessary step. Our focus is on the first step of healing Hashimoto's by addressing the gut... which we will discuss in the next chapter.

Testing – Always test before taking your thyroid medication (if you are on medication). Taking thyroid medication before the lab test can falsely elevate your thyroid status for a few hours.

Thyroid Markers

TSH – Thyroid Stimulating Hormone is a hormone released by the pituitary gland. It senses whether or not you have circulating levels of low or high thyroid hormone. In advanced cases of Hashimoto's and primary hypothyroidism, the TSH is going to be elevated. We cannot rely only on TSH, as this hormone fluctuates in the blood.

T4 and T3 are the two main thyroid hormones. Total hormone levels measure all of the thyroid hormones in the body. Free hormone levels measure the hormone that is available to do its job in the body.

Free T4 – T4 is the storage hormone. Free means you are measuring what is available and unbound.

Free T3 – T3 is the active thyroid hormone. Free means you are measuring what is available and unbound. If your free T3 is high, you could have Hashimoto's. If your free T3 is mid-range or lower, you may have hypothyroidism.

Reverse T3 – Reverse T3 (rT3) is an inactive form of T3. The T4 can be converted to either T3 or reverse T3. It's biologically normal for some of your T4 to convert to rT3 and some to T3, yet the amount that translates to rT3, which is not available for metabolic function, can become excessive in cases of chronic stress. This is a marker that reflects peripheral thyroid metabolism; not so much what the thyroid is making, but what the body is doing with what the thyroid is making.

Thyroglobulin Antibodies (TgAb) – Measures the level of the antibody protein antithyroglobulin in order to discern the presence of Hashimoto's. Antibodies are proteins in your immune system that serve to identify and remove foreign antigens. Thyroglobulin is a protein that exists solely within your thyroid gland to synthesize T4 and T3 hormones.

Thyroid Peroxidase (TPO) are proteins in your immune system that serve to identify and remove foreign antigens. Peroxidase is an enzyme that is critical in the conversion of T4 to T3. TPO is a key measurement in the detection of Hashimoto's.

Self Exam Screen:

> You need a mirror and a glass of water. Examine the area just below the Adam's apple and look for anything asymmetrical. Next, lift your chin up and drink some water while looking in the mirror. If you notice any area that protrudes or sticks out, talk to your doctor and let him or her examine it.

An ultrasound is a noninvasive test that can be very helpful and is underutilized. Thyroid cancer is the fastest-increasing type of cancer in North America today. Tissue changes begin years before it develops into cancer. Being able to intercept this process before it becomes cancer can save a life. There is no radiation and there is no side effect. If they are abnormal, it is good to track at least once per year. If there are lesions growing, at least every six months.

Do I need Medication?

Most of our patients say, "Doc, I just don't want to be on medication the rest of my life." Here are the 3 times that medication is absolutely necessary:

- **History of thyroid cancer**
- **Complete thyroidectomy**
- **Gland has been destroyed**

People may benefit from Thyroid Medications if

- Elevated TSH, suppressed T4
- Thyroid nodules or goitrous findings
- TSH > 2

It's important to understand that you may also use thyroid medication such as Nature-Throid or Westhroid as a bridge. We can start with smaller doses until the lifestyle and behavioral changes kick in and you no longer need it.

5 stages of Hashimoto's

Stage 1

Genetic predisposition – see no evidence.

Stage 2

Immune cell infiltration into thyroid gland – may see autoimmune markers.

Stage 3

Subclinical hypothyroidism.

Stage 4

Overt hypothyroidism

Increased TSH. Decreased T3. Decreased T4 (diagnosis stage).

Stage 5

Progression to other autoimmune disorders.

Other Signs and Clues:

Long before laboratory testing shows tissue changes, practitioners trained in Ayruvedic or Traditional Chinese Medicine have used the ancient wisdom of interpreting the body signals through changes in the fingernails, the tongue, wrist pulse, and eyes.

Fingernail Diagnosis – Vertical ridges on the nails may be the result of imbalanced nourishment – excess carbohydrate and salt intake. The digestive, liver, and kidney functions may be underactive and the person may have general fatigue.

White dots on the nails – Shows the elimination of sugars. Can also represent zinc deficiency.

Split Nails – Chaotic diet. The circulatory, reproductive, and nervous systems are in disorder.

"Every cell in the body has receptor sites for thyroid hormones. Thyroid hormones are responsible for the most basic and fundamental aspect of physiology, the basal metabolic rate. Lack of ideal thyroid hormone leads to global decline in cellular function of all bodily systems. The thyroid is the central gear in the complex web of metabolism and extremely sensitive to minor imbalances in other areas of physiology. An astute clinician should always ask what else is going wrong, as a result and cause, when he or she identifies a thyroid imbalance."

—Datis Kharrazian, DHSc, DC, MS, MNeuroScience

Stick your tongue out takes on new meaning when you consider the following tongue diagnosis

Which tongue are you?

A healthy tongue is pink without ridges, cracks or swollen.

Examine your tongue. Go ahead and look in the mirror.

A swollen tongue may indicate bloating or fullness in the chest or abdomen. In Traditional Chinese medicine it is thought to have excess "dampness" in the body.

Thin white coating on the tongue is associated with unstable emotional state, stress and/or depression.

Cracks and redness are associated with hot flushes, ringing in the ears and symptoms of menopause

Pale tongue without coating may be associated with dizziness, poor concentration, insomnia and fatigue

Red tongue with thin yellow coating is associated with constipation, skin problems and feeling hot all over

Purple tongue with black spots – painful legs, headaches, cold limbs and varicose veins

Pale swollen tongue with thick white coating – associated with back pain, tendency to panic, impotence/infertility, feel cold easily

Chapter summary

- ✓ Get the proper testing done even if you have to pay out of pocket
- ✓ Consider a baseline Thyroid Ultrasound
- ✓ Find a practitioner that is skilled in Autonomic Response Testing – Find Your Root Cause
- ✓ Do a self exam every month-When to medicate
- ✓ 4 stages of Hashimoto's
- ✓ Other signs and clues
- ✓ Which tongue are you?

Your Living Gut

In this chapter we will have a paradigm shift in how you think about your gut. Up until your diagnosis you may not have given it much attention. We'll see that healing begins with an "intention," but what will make the difference is where you place your "attention."

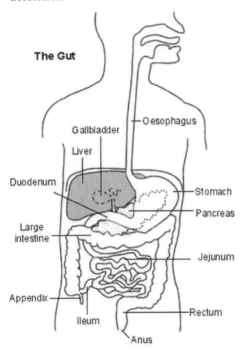

The Gut

Oesophagus
Gallbladder
Liver
Duodenum
Stomach
Pancreas
Large intestine
Jejunum
Appendix
Rectum
Ileum
Anus

We can think of the gut as a hollow tube that runs from the mouth to the anus.

It's a living ecosystem. It is a 22-foot long living ecosystem.

Think about it this way: Imagine you want to drive cross-country from New Jersey to California. The journey from one coast to another coast will differ for you depending on whether you choose a motorcycle or a badass truck. Will you be staying in luxury hotels or

27

backpacking in hostels? Will you be dining in fine restaurants or eating fast food? Will you use a GPS to navigate, or an outdated road map?

Two people with the same goal will have very different experiences.

This is same way to think about your living gut. Those born through the birth canal vs C-section and those breastfed instead of formula fed will cultivate and develop very different ecosystems.

While we all may be eating, digesting, metabolizing, and pooping and peeing, the journey the nutrients take will be very different, and what may or may not be absorbed and excreted can be extremely different. This is what gut health is all about.

My husband and I have similar cultural backgrounds with grandparents all migrating from Italy. We grew up with similar lifestyles, and for the first 11 years of our lives went to the same elementary school. Yet, I often giggle and call him a goat because he can eat nearly any type of food at any time and have perfect digestion, metabolism, and excretion. I, on the other hand, have to follow pretty much a Paleo – Autoimmune Paleo diet, with careful attention placed on the quality of the food, who prepared it, and what mood I am when I am eating it. Otherwise I can end up with bloat, constipation, and fatigue.

One of the big differences between my husband and me was that he grew up on fermented foods. When you think about the gut as a living ecosystem not unlike the rain forest, which needs a different soil composition, adequate hydration, proper ratio of enzymatic processes and sunlight, our living gut needs the same. Fermented foods contain live bacteria that function as natural probiotics. My husband said there was always sauerkraut in the house and he put it on everything. His grandmother would tell him how good it was for the gut, and in the Old Country every family made their own from scratch, including yogurt and pickled vegetables.

Each culture seems to have their favorites, from kimchi, to kefir and lassi, to sauerkraut. Processed food does not contain any live cultures – in fact, some would argue whether it really qualifies as food. We have been brainwashed by commercial ads showing succulent foods that encourage us to get off the couch to eat a pizza, run out for Happy Meal, or get more energy with a Red Bull. Sadly, these commercials have us thinking this is NATURAL, and we believe this is FOOD.

It is not. Food does not come in a box, it grows on a tree. It is not found in a microwavable plastic tray, it is found on a bush. It does not drip out of a nozzle from a WaWa, it comes from a natural spring. Food is found on vines, in the soil, hanging on a bush, swimming in the sea or running on the earth. FOOD DOES NOT GROW IN A BOX.

If you were born through the vaginal canal you are off to a better start than someone who was not, but that is only the beginning. This rich microbiome has to be cultivated. How does this happen?

In an ideal scenario, before your mother became a mom, she began to enrich her own ecosystem. She ate a whole food diet, removed her amalgams, didn't smoke or drink, and had little exposure to electromagnetic fields such as power lines, wi-fi, and cell phones. She also dealt with her unhealed emotional and family traumas and loved your father unconditionally. Same for your dad.

Her pregnancy was filled with joy, nourishment, proper micro and macro nutrients, and she felt supported and safe.

You were born in a birthing center or at home with natural lighting, uplifting music, and gentle touch. You came through the birth canal, and there you received not only her bacterial imprint carrying life-giving healthy bacterial codes and information, but you also received a rich download of cultural and generational colonies of mutualistic and commensal organisms.

Mutualistic organisms are ones that benefit both themselves and the host. Commensal organisms benefit either themselves or the host without hurting the other, while parasitic organisms cause harm to the host.

This download you received if you came through the birth canal is then cultivated, developed, and nourished if you were breast fed and later given wholesome foods and pure water and protected from environmental toxins such as insecticides and chemicals.

Sadly, this picture does NOT represent the majority of us.

Today one in three children is born by Caesarian section. They are already compromised by not having received the life-giving probiotics from a vaginal birth. Why are there so many Caesarian births? That's another book.

The lining of our gut is comprised of cells that are tightly stacked on to each other. It's designed this way so that as food passes through the gut, the cells can absorb the good micro and macro nutrients and eliminate what isn't good through the urine or feces. When these tightly stacked cells become separated we call that "leaky gut."

Perhaps you have found yourself to be gluten intolerant or know someone who is. My 11-year-old grandson was visiting last summer, and I noticed he spent a lot of time in the bathroom for a young boy. We would be out riding bicycles and he would often yell, "Nonni, I have to find a bathroom right away!"

I noticed he was always grabbing for tissue for his runny nose, and despite his active sport life he just couldn't get rid of that little tummy. I began to keep a watchful eye on what he was eating and how he reacted. His mornings were often a bagel followed by pasta for lunch or dinner, and a treat of some sugary confection. I began to point out to him how his body was reacting to these foods and he began to take notice. He decided to do an experiment and voluntarily removed these foods and observed the changes.

After 2 weeks of being gluten free he called me with a most chipper voice. "Nonni... I haven't had diarrhea for 2 weeks and I am not going through a box of tissues a day anymore! I feel great," he said. I began to talk to him about his courage to take on a culture of fast foods and quick fixes and how little support children get from their peers. Going to other kids' parties is filled with landmines of sugar and gluten-laden foods. I was trying to tell him how proud I was of him and his response really surprised me. He said, "I have other friends who have gone gluten free, so I don't feel alone, and I really like feeling better, so I don't miss it." Wow.

We'll talk more about about the gluten thing in *Sick to my Gut*.

98% of our immune system is found within the gut. Please reread that sentence. It is not only true, but it is critical to being well and staying well and getting well.

Let's pause to remember our anatomy. The thyroid gland is a part of the Endocrine system. Notice the relationship between the thyroid and the stomach, adrenal gland and liver.

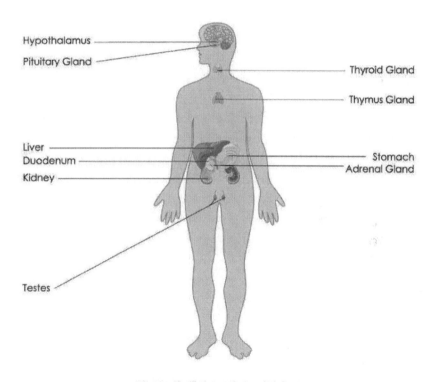

ENDOCRINE SYSTEM

Did you know we have way more bacteria in our gut than we do cells in our body? They are part of the information highway driving the neuronal connections. This superhighway is designed to be initiated when we are born through the vaginal canal and continues to evolve throughout life.

My paternal grandparents were born in Italy and migrated to USA when they were in their early 30's. The first step they took was to plant a garden and make a wine cellar. Growing up next door to them, I grew accustomed to the sight of grapes being churned and lush lettuce and tomatoes being harvested from the garden. This garden not only fed my grandparents, but my family and my neighboring cousins as well.

I would often find my grandfather in the garden and he would tell me to look for earthworms. He seemed so happy when the soil contained many of these slimy creatures. Like many good farmers and gardeners, he knew earthworms dig tunnels deep in the garden bed that allows for roots of the plants to be nourished, and when they pooped they left behind phosphorus, calcium, nitrogen, and magnesium that help to produce nutrient-rich crops. Have you ever wondered why farmers love to have lots of varieties of manure added to their soil? This is nature's first probiotic. Since the 1970s, there have been soil microbes for sale in the garden shop, and in 2014, the global biofertilizers market size was estimated at USD 535.8 million.

Though we never see them, ninety percent of all organisms on the seven continents live underground. In addition to bacteria and fungi, the soil is also filled with protozoa, nematodes, mites, and microarthropods. There can be 10,000 to 50,000 species in less than a teaspoon of soil. In that same teaspoon of soil, there are more microbes than there are people on the earth. In a handful of healthy soil, there is more biodiversity in just the bacterial community than you will find in all the animals of the Amazon basin.

Thus the microbial community in the soil, like in the human biome, provides "invasion resistance" services to its symbiotic partner. As author of *In Defense of Food*, Michael Pollan, recently noted, "Some researchers believe that the alarming increase in autoimmune diseases in the West may owe to a disruption in the ancient relationship between our bodies and their 'old friends' – the microbial symbionts with whom we co-evolved."

In 2008, the National Institutes of Health launched the Human Microbiome Project (a counterpart to the Human Genome Project). The primary objective was to study how the trillions of microbes in and around our body affect it.The second phase of the project is looking at the relationship between the microbiome and "diseases of interest," which would include autoimmune conditions. The NIH project is one of seven international microbiome research efforts to understand the human microbiome.

The Microbiome – Our Inner Garden

Our bodies are thought to be home to about 10 bacterial cells for every human cell, but they're so small that together microbes make up about 1 percent to 3 percent of someone's body mass. Those bacterial genes produce substances that perform specific jobs, some of which play critical roles in the health and development of their human hosts, said Dr. Bruce Birren of the Broad Institute of MIT and Harvard, another of the project's investigators. Genes from gut bacteria, for example, lead to digestion of certain proteins and fats. They also produce certain beneficial compounds, like inflammation-fighting chemicals.

Already the findings are reshaping scientists' views of how people stay healthy, or not.

"This is a whole new way of looking at human biology and human disease, and it's awe-inspiring," said Dr. Phillip Tarr of Washington University at St. Louis, one of the lead researchers in the $173 million project, funded by the National Institutes of Health.

"These bacteria are not passengers," Tarr stressed. "They are metabolically active. As a community, we now have to reckon with them like we have to reckon with the ecosystem in a forest or a body of water."

And like environmental ecosystems, your microbial makeup varies widely by body part. Your skin could be like a rainforest, your intestines teeming with different species like an ocean.

They live on your skin, up your nose, in your gut – enough bacteria, fungi, and other microbes that if collected together could weigh, amazingly, a few pounds.

One surprise: It turns out that nearly everybody harbors low levels of some harmful types of bacteria, pathogens that are known for causing specific infections. But when a person is healthy – like the 242 U.S. adults who volunteered to be tested for the project – those bugs simply quietly coexist with benign or helpful microbes, perhaps kept in check by them.

The next step is to explore what doctors really want to know: Why do the bad bugs harm some people and not others? What changes a person's microbial zoo that puts them at risk? There are about 22,000 human genes. But the microbes add to our bodies the power of many, many more – about 8 million genes, the new project estimated.

Also, researchers at Baylor College of Medicine reported that the kind of bacteria living in the vagina changes during pregnancy, perhaps to give the fetus as healthy a passage as possible. Previous research has found differences in what bacteria babies first absorb, depending on whether they're born vaginally or by C-section, a possible explanation for why Caesareans raise the risk for certain infections.

All of this new information in some ways is humbling, because it shows how much more work is needed to understand this world within us, noted infectious disease specialist Dr. David Relman of Stanford University, who wrote a review of the project's findings for the journal *Nature*.

This living gut also needs a proper pH to thrive. Perhaps you have heard discussions on alkaline versus acidic. This is controlled by stomach acids. These acids are essential in digesting protein and protecting us from invaders such as *H. pylori* and *E. coli*. Just like a proper pH in a swimming pool or fish tank is vital to the life of the organisms or fish, so is the pH of our gut vital to the microbiome.

Along with adequate hydration, the right food and rest and exercise, and certain minerals such as zinc, are essential to maintaining the proper pH. Most Hashimoto patients have low Alkaline Phosphatase, which leads to deficient zinc and low stomach acid. People who rely on products such as Nexium, Tagamet, Zantac, and Prilosec may be creating a host of additional problems such as vitamin B12 deficiency. Gluten contributes to both acid reflux and vitamin B12 deficiency, only compounding an already smoldering problem.

In the chapter on *Gut Solutions,* we'll talk about ways to assess and support proper stomach pH.

Many times patients are on medications that are known to contribute to leaky gut, such as corticosteroids: Steroid drugs such as prednisone suppress the immune system and dampen inflammation. While they may be life-saving or necessary, they also can contribute to leaky gut. This is because they raise cortisol, which in high doses breaks down the gut lining. This is why chronic stress, which also raises cortisol, contributes to leaky gut as well.

Non-steroidal anti-inflammatory drugs (NSAIDs): NSAIDs such as ibuprofen and aspirin have been shown to increase intestinal permeability within 24 hours of use, and long-term use can contribute to a leaky gut condition.

Antibiotics: Antibiotics wipe out the beneficial gut flora, which can lead to leaky gut. It's important to always follow up antibiotic use with probiotics to re-inoculate the gut.

Chemotherapy drugs: Chemotherapy drugs can lead to leaky gut by degrading the intestinal barrier.

While these drugs may be necessary at times, we must remain vigilant in understanding the consequences and protecting against them.

Chapter Summary:

- ✓ Food does not come in a box
- ✓ The gut is a living, 22-foot ecosystem
- ✓ We are inoculated at birth through the vaginal canal
- ✓ 98% of your immune system is in the gut
- ✓ No two people have the same gut microbiome – it's as unique as your fingerprint
- ✓ We need a proper pH to thrive
- ✓ Antibiotics and other medications wipe out beneficial flora
- ✓ Being gluten-free is a must. Just don't replace it with other "processed" gluten free products

Sick to my gut

When patients come in they usually have an idea as to what they want. They tell us they want more energy, to be pain free, or to feel good again. What they need us for is they have usually done a host of treatments and remedies, and some have helped and others not at all, but the bottom line is they still feel they are missing the root cause. A big question mark is when to begin detoxification. Often patients have done a variety of detoxification program and their symptoms only worsened because toxins just recirculated. The gut is the main elimination organ. When you begin with the gut, most detoxification programs will be more efficient and have greater results.

As a visual learner it's helpful for me to see the big picture. This flowchart shows the multiple pathways involved in the process of dis-ease from early triggers to later diagnosis.

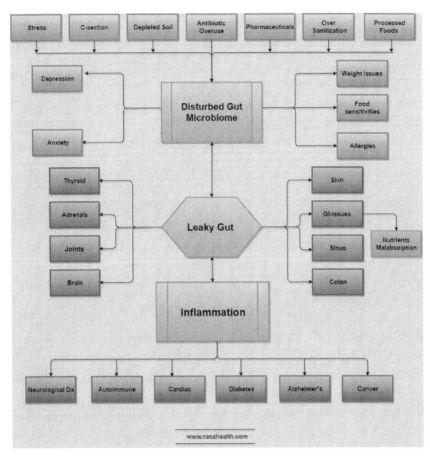

Take a moment and review the above diagram. You can see the many factors and pathways involved, but I want to draw your attention to the "inflammation." A February 2004 issue of *Time* magazine had an article called "*Inflammation – The Silent Killer.*"

On the outer membrane of certain bacteria found in the gut is a combination of sugars and fats that are called Lipopolysaccharide, or LPS for short. This LPS is there to protect bacteria from being digested by bile salts secreted by the gallbladder. The LPS is doing its job when it lives where it belongs. However, when the gut becomes "leaky," this LPS is able to pass into systemic circulation, where it triggers a violent inflammatory response.

As it turns out, there are a number of ways we can feel "sick to our guts." Lining the small intestine are tiny cells that form together much like Legos and make up "tight junctions."

They are there to not only absorb the right nutrients, but they are designed to block foreign or undigested foods from reaching the bloodstream. When these cells become separated, we call this "leaky gut," or dysbiosis. A leaky gut leads to inflammation and potential autoimmunity when the tight gap junctions, also called Zonula Occludens, allow for Zonulans (small proteins) to wedge themselves between the passageways and allow foreign substances to make their way into the bloodstream. Substances like gluten increase the production of those Zonulan proteins, causing more of those tight gap junctions to become permeable, leading to inflammation, autoimmunity, and even cancer.

Leaky Gut

Signs of Leaky Gut

- Food allergies or food sensitivities
- Autoimmune disorders, fibromyalgia, chronic fatigue syndrome or lupus
- Bloating, gas, constipation, loose stools, heartburn and nutrient malabsorption
- Inflammatory Bowel Disease (IBD), including, IBS Crohn's or colitis
- Thyroid issues such as hypothyroidism, Hashimoto's thyroiditis or Graves disease
- Adrenal fatigue, candida and slow metabolism
- Anxiety, depression and autism
- Joint and and muscle pain
- Many skin problems: eczema, psoriasis, rosacea, acne and age spots

A healthy digestive tract breaks down foods into small particles and releases these beneficial nutrients into the bloodstream. When the gut is not healthy and becomes too permeable, it becomes difficult to digest foods. Some of the most common offenders are gluten casein and soy. This can affect the body by:

- Impairing the ability to absorb valuable nutrients
- Triggering autoimmune reactions
- Improper elimination of toxins from the body, which can affect brain function

One of the big culprits with leaky gut is gluten. As of 2012, it was estimated that 18 million Americans have gluten sensitivity. Gluten is a protein contained in the grains of wheat, barley, rye, and oats. This protein gives the doughy, elastic consistency to flours used to make bread. There are 2 big schools of thought as to why this protein is wreaking havoc with our guts.

Here's the first. Remember we talked about those cells in our gut that are stacked closely together? They have a structure known as "villi." These villi are tiny hair-like follicles that absorb nutrients. They are responsible for providing the transport mechanism from the tube, from the small intestine into the body. Approximately 90% of what we eat is assimilated by those villi. In the 60's we had "shag" carpeting. Every time you walked on the shag carpeting, the tiny hairs would flatten and lose their puffiness and piling. The only way to get them back would be to vacuum the shag. In our guts, these tiny villi become pummeled by toxins, or excess mucus, which can be caused by a sensitivity to gluten, or dairy, or soy – even infection and pathogens. When these villi become damaged we can no longer absorb the nutrients, which not only lead to major nutrient deficiencies, but weight gain or loss as well. Why? The feedback signal to the brain is carrying the message "there is a famine coming...store fat."

All grains contain some form of gluten. The most common reaction patients have when we find a gluten sensitivity is, "HOW CAN WHEAT BE BAD FOR ME... my family was raised on pasta, bread and flour and they all lived long and healthy lives."

"I'm glad you asked," I tell them. See, people in America with a gluten sensitivity will often travel to Europe and eat many gluten-filled meals and never suffer a bit. What is the difference?

While wheat has been consumed for thousands of years in kernel form and ground fresh, today's wheat is making people sick. Modern industrial milling is fast and efficient, but the product isn't the same. This process influences how the kernel is separated and allows for a "barren" flour. Many other processes of the Green Revolution of the mid 1900's gave rise to high-yielding varieties of grains that could be shipped over long distances, but left us with a lesser grain. Add the new synthetic fertilizers, hybridized seeds, and chemical pesticides that saw regular use.

The second big reason is the effects of insecticides such as Round Up.

Enter glyphosate. Glyphosate is the active ingredient found in Round Up – America's #1 weed killer. It seems that no one is asking the question: if it is so effective at killing the weeds, what else is it killing? According to Dr. Stephanie Seneff, a senior research scientist at the Massachusetts Institute of Technology (MIT), glyphosate appears to be strongly correlated with not only gluten disorders, but autism, infertility, and many chronic diseases. I first heard Dr. Seneff present at the 2015 Healing Your Brain Conference in New Jersey. It was one of those lectures that left you feeling sick to your stomach and angry at the feeling of helplessness that ensued.

Europe does not permit the use of glyphosate. Is this one of the reasons gluten sensitive people can eat gluten when traveling abroad?

According to Dr. Seneff's research, the glyphosate is destroying the villi we discussed earlier, which reduces our ability to absorb vitamins and minerals. The good bacteria in our gut are dependent on these nutrients to flourish and thrive. This contributes to the imbalance in our gut ecosystem, leading to irritable bowel syndrome, constipation, bloating, leaky gut, and autoimmune disease as well.

Anything that goes in the mouth and isn't digested will pass right out the other end. Everything that happens inside this hollow tube has to do with digestion, absorption, and elimination.

Leptin

Leptin is a hormone made by fat cells that was only discovered in 1994. It is sometimes referred to as the "fat hormone." It sends a signal to the brain to say we have enough stored energy and that we don't need to eat. Sometimes that signal doesn't get through, so we eat and fat gets stored, and fat cells secrete more leptin. It is similar to insulin resistance. Leptin has a strong bearing on how much thyroid hormone is produced by your thyroid gland.

Eating too much can lead us to become "leptin resistant." When leptin resistance happens in the body, it basically 'tells' your thyroid gland via complex signaling hormones to slow down metabolism and stop burning food for calories. In other words, it tells you to hold on to fat to survive the famine (remember it thinks you are starving to death).

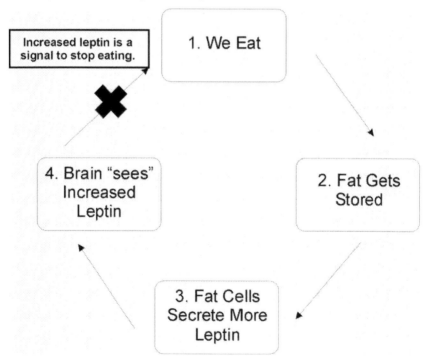

Leptin resistance = Fat storage

Leptin resistance drives obesity by inflaming the thyroid gland. As leptin levels (and leptin resistance) increase, your body starts to turn T4 into Reverse T3 in an attempt to slow down metabolism (because it thinks you're starving).

Serum leptin levels should be <12. Another indicator is a high uric acid level. Anything >5 is a strong predictor for developing obesity, diabetes, insulin resistance, and fatty liver.

We treat leptin resistance much the same way that insulin resistance is treated: diet and exercise. High-intensity interval training and intermittent fasting.

Blood Sugar

About 50% of people with Hashimoto's have tested for high blood sugar or impaired glucose metabolism. Things like brain fog, anxiety, palpitations, night sweats, thinning hair, and headaches can all be related to blood sugar imbalances, as well as infertility, chronic fungal infections, and PCOS.

Diet makes a big difference here. Limiting refined carbohydrates and potatoes and getting plenty of good fats and proteins throughout the day can be helpful. One of my favorite herbs for balancing blood sugar is Berberine.

Balancing Blood Sugar Rules

- Never skip breakfast
- Include fat/protein with every meal
- Avoid fruit juice
- Avoid all grains, dairy, corn, soy, and wheat
- Limit caffeine
- No foods with a glycemic index > 55

Candida

Candida albicans is a single-celled fungus that is normally present in the gastrointestinal and genitourinary tracts. In normal, healthy individuals, these yeasts are kept in balance by beneficial bacteria. When the internal terrain becomes compromised, Candida organisms grow out of control and cause infection. One of the big problems is that this yeast gives off many toxins, like zymosan, which causes inflammation. Many people notice that their symptoms become exacerbated after exposure to damp and moldy places.

This overgrowth must be controlled because it can lead to a systemic candidiasis when the yeast travels through the blood to infect every organ of the body.

Over 90% of a healthy population is "allergic" to candida, so we often see hives, asthma, eczema, chronic vaginitis, abdominal cramps, and diarrhea which has its roots in a candida issue.

The solution is to starve the yeast, and we can do this with a yeast free, sugar-free diet, along with antifungal supplements as well as re-inoculating the gut with healthy probiotics.

Infections:

Hashimoto's is a combination of genetic predisposition, food sensitivities, nutrient deficiencies, adrenal issues, and gut imbalances, as well as toxins and infections both bacterial and viral. Each of these do not stand alone, but in fact have a direct or indirect impact on each other.

Working through each layer can seem overwhelming at first. We begin with the gut because you are also impacting every other layer and laying the foundation for deeper and more refined treatment that the body will greatly respond to.

Some of the more common infections we find in Hashimoto's are Blastocystis hominis and h-pylori and giardia. While a great diet can help to boost the immune system, it is often not enough to eradicate the underlying infections. Each infection requires a different treatment to be most effective. These are best identified through proper testing and treatment by a knowledgeable holistic, integrated, and functional medicine practitioner.

Biofilm

When you go to the dentist for a cleaning the Hygienist is removing excess plaque, or "biofilm." Just as there are healthy and unhealthy bacteria, we also find that we can have healthy and unhealthy biofilm. Beneficial microflora create a thin mucus – biofilm – that allows the passage of nutrients through the intestinal wall that is moistening, lubricating, and anti-inflammatory. The colon has a mucous layer to prevent any bacteria infiltrating the underlying epithelial cells.

It is possible that people with decreased mucosal integrity are at risk for bacteria to invade and form these biofilms, which may eventually lead to cancer. In fact, according to one study, people with an unhealthy biofilm formation in their colon have a 5-fold increase in their likelihood to get colorectal cancer, much higher than any other known indicator.

An unhealthy gut biofilm promotes inflammation and is difficult to penetrate when trying to treat an underlying infection. It also prevents the full absorption of nutrients across the intestinal wall.

Recommendation:

Proteolytic enzymes – Proteolytic enzymes can help to break apart the structure of unhealthy gut biofilm when taken on an empty stomach. Proteolytic enzymes are enzymes like protease, papain, and peptidases. Look for the highest quality.

We also use CPTG (certified pure therapeutic grade) essential oils, which I will address in *Gut Solutions.*

Lyme Disease

We often find patients with Hashimoto's to be positive for Borrelia Burgdorferi or one of the common co-infections like Babesia and/or Bartonella.

45

Mold toxicity

When taking patient histories, we often find there has been a past and/or recent exposure to mold, and a patient who is still being exposed will not get better until the exposure is removed.

Heavy metals

This must be assessed and treated accordingly.

Genetic Testing

Testing for the MTHFR gene mutation can be helpful. I would also like to comment that this is the "new kid on the block." Patients will come in with their labs showing polymorphisms and often they feel as though they are a victim of their genes. This is simply not so. We now understand that it is the "epigenetics" that runs the show. These are factors that turn the gene on or off. Simply having the gene is NOT enough. Having the information may be helpful in understanding possible treatment effectiveness but it is not, in my opinion, how we approach a case or even define treatment

Many people have methylation factors that predispose us to certain outcomes. It can contribute to inflammation and reduce the body's ability to eliminate toxins. People who have this gene mutation don't utilize folic acid properly, which can lead to a folate deficiency. We recommend methylated or active folate for our patients who have the MTHFR gene mutation.

Epstein Barr – In addition to gut infections, we also see dental issues and sinusitis through the bystander effect. Epstein-Barr has been associated with many autoimmune diseases including lupus and Hashimoto's.

Treating infections is beyond the scope of this book, but viral infections, stealth infections, Lyme disease, mold, and Epstein Barr should be considered by every patient diagnosed with Hashimoto's Disease. While the gut will never be fully healed until we address the underlying infections the solutions outlined in this book will be a huge step in beginning the process.

SIBO

Small intestinal bacterial overgrowth

This is quite common in people with Hypothyroidism. It is an overgrowth of bacteria in the small intestine, a place it should not be. SIBO is a big contributor to leaky gut and intestinal permeability. Symptoms can include bloating, flatulence, abdominal discomfort, constipation, and/or diarrhea. Some patients who have tested positive have not reported any symptoms. People with SIBO tend to have low ferritin, and people respond well to Oil of Oregano two or three times per day. Allicillin has also been effective. These people must avoid Gluten!

Recommendations:

Check B12 levels, Vitamin D, and iron levels.

The GAPS diet and Low FODMAPS can be very helpful.

Recommended Tests:

www.stoolanalyzer.com

Biohealth 401 H – Biohealth Labs – helpful to identify gut infections

GI Effects Profile – Metametrix – helpful with gut bacteria

Cyrex Array #2 – www.cyrexlabs.com – Leaky Gut

Autonomic Response Testing – Find a practitioner certified in this technique www.klinghardtacademy.com (can be used to both identify the bacteria, toxin, infection, parasite and/or treatment

Chapter summary

- ✓ Consider the root cause. One system impacts another
- ✓ Get assessed for leaky gut and then fix it
- ✓ Treat the gut before you begin detoxification
- ✓ Get tested for Leptins- Balance your Blood sugar
- ✓ Detoxify from glyphosate
- ✓ Test for underlying pathogens and infections
- ✓ SIBO has special requirements
- ✓ Consider methylation issues but recognize epigenetics run the show
- ✓ Heavy metal testing

It's a Gut Feeling

Have you heard yourself say these words? "I feel it in my gut?" As it turns out, there is scientific evidence that explains not only is this possible, but it is one way the body communicates with us.

Patients are often surprised when I tell them early fetal development of the brain and the gut originate from the same type of embryonic tissue. When this tissue divides, one part develops into your central nervous system (brain and spinal cord) and the other become the tube that goes from your mouth to your gut, also known as the Enteric Nervous System.

Because of the similar neuronal structure, the Enteric Nervous System (ENS) is referred to as The Second Brain or the brain in the belly.

In later stages of development, these two similar structures become united by the VAGUS NERVE. The Vagus Nerve is the longest nerve in our body and directly connects our brain and our gut. It is along this nerve that messages and signals are both sent and received from the brain to the gut. This is an essential communication lifeline and can make a big difference as to whether we get sick or not.

Infections along this path can affect how the messages are sent. Salmonella infections have been shown to affect activity, as well as Staphylococcus.

What happens in Vagus doesn't always stay in Vagus

In a study with mice, a probiotic bacteria, Lactobacillus Rhamnous, showed a direct impact on neurotransmitter receptors in the Central Nervous System (CNS). Serotonin is one neurotransmitter found in the gut that regulates mood, sleep, and learning, and also plays a major role in digestion. Serotonin signaling from the gut to the head alerts the brain to activity in the gut and has led to a new term, our "PsychoBiome." Our psychobiome helps us understand how the bacteria in the gut are like little factories producing key neurotransmitters: GABA, Norepinephrine, Dopamine, and how the metabolic actions of these bacteria impact the fatty acid composition of the brain.

In the above study, Lactobacillus Rhamnous had a direct impact on GABA, the main inhibitory transmitter involved in regulating many physiological and psychological processes. When this Vagus nerve in the mice was cut (vagotomized) the neurochemical and behavioral effects were not found. These findings highlight the important role of bacteria in the bidirectional communication of the gut-brain axis and suggests that certain organisms may prove to be useful therapeutic agents in stress-related disorders such as anxiety and depression.

What's bugging you?

Could it be that our state of mind and the path to happiness is less likely to be found in the self-help section of the bookstore, but is more likely to be found within your own microbiome?

Kelly Brogan, MD, is a holistic psychiatrist who has made a lot of waves in the conventional treatment of depression and mental illness with her holistic approach. In *"A Mind of Your own"* Kelly lists some new ideas when dealing with mental health and depression:

- Prevention is possible
- Medication treatment comes at a steep cost
- Optimal health is not possible through education
- Your health is under your control
- Working with lifestyle medicine – simple everyday habits that don't entail drugs – is a safe and effective way to send the body a signal of safety

Because of this direct gut-brain connection, we can see how our gut has a huge impact on our physical, emotional, and cognitive abilities. When we find excessive bad bacteria, we often find obsessive compulsive disorders, mood swings, anxiety, and depression.

Let's look at this through the digestive process. There are four steps to digestion.

- Cephalic
- Esophageal
- Gastric
- Intestinal

Cephalic

The first one is something we hear least about, and I feel it is the step that has compromised us most. The first phase of Cephalic digestion has everything to do with how we think about food, shop for our food, prepare our food, and the smell of food.

One of my go-to options for my chronically ill patients is to begin with broths. Broths can be complex, with many types of bones, or simply prepared from an assortment of vegetables. The biggest obstacle for many is finding the time to prepare it. My patients tell me they would rather buy store-bought or have someone else make if for them.

This is where I have to explain the "Cephalic" phase of digestion and why they will be missing this key step when they opt not to shop, prepare, and cook it themselves. Of course, there are times when we choose to eat out, and that is fine, but what I'm talking about here is the importance of this phase of digestion. Think about it. When a snowy blizzard is on its way, are you more apt to want a warm stew or soup brewing on the stove with the rich smell of dill or rosemary filling your home with their aromas? A home has to "smell" like a home. The smells of onions and garlic and cookies and vanilla can have such an impact on our digestion and emotions that any good realtor knows the best way to stage a home for sale is to put some cookies in the oven. Have you noticed the smell of cinnamon when stepping into your favorite grocery store? They do this because the science shows how smell impacts our behavior, and now we understand how it impacts our digestion.

Praying over our food or taking a moment of gratitude is an important part of the Cephalic phase of digestion. In Middle Eastern cultures, critical attention is placed on the atmosphere and ambiance of the dining room. Soothing colors and quiet sounds are preferred over the Western approach of multiple television sets competing for your attention and the music so loud it is impossible to have a conversation. Eating your lunch behind the steering wheel after a drive through is called a "happy meal" in the US, while other cultures would consider it death.

Esophageal

Once we swallow food it enters the esophagus. In many of the chronic and autoimmune conditions we see today, patients often complain that they just can't "swallow." This important phase is designed to keep the stomach acids from coming back up into the mouth. This function can be impacted by low stomach acid or a very acidic pH. Remember, it is the stomach acid that is our first defence against unfriendly pathogens like parasites and other critters. When the stomach acid is low it also impacts our B-12 levels, resulting in different kinds of anemia or SIBO (small intestinal bacterial overgrowth).

Gastric

During the gastric phase of digestion, the muscles of your stomach wall flex to help mix together food particles, gastric juice, and pepsin, a protein-digesting enzyme secreted by your stomach that breaks protein chains in smaller pieces called peptides. Digestive enzymes with pepsin can be very helpful here.

Some simple ways to invite stomach acid are taking lemon in water or raw apple cider vinegar.

Intestinal Phase

Remember those villi we talked about earlier? This is where 90% of what we eat is assimilated through those finger-like projections. This happens in the small intestine where the food particles are separated into nutrients and waste. This is where the proper micro and macro nutrients are absorbed that will feed and fuel our cells. When those villi have become damaged and compromised from food sensitivities or medications, they can lead to intestinal inflammation, degeneration, and nutrient depletion. Now the stage is set for leaky gut and Candida to occur, and these are two conditions that easily lead to a Hashimoto's diagnosis if combined with predisposed genes and toxins and/or infections. Taking thyroid medicine does nothing to correct this imbalance.

What's your Gut Type?

The biggest question on new patients' minds is, "What can I eat?" Food is so essential for not only nourishment, but our emotional and cultural self as well. When considering the best "diet" for a patient, many factors must be considered, and each patient is considered for their unique story, genetics, culture, and digestive health. We try to consider each patient according to their gut type as explained by Dr. Josh Axe in his book *"Eat Dirt"*.

Five Gut Types

1. Immune
2. Stressed
3. Gastric
4. Toxic
5. Candida

We'll address them in the chapter on *Gut Solutions*

Who's *Buggin'* You?

When considering the root cause for Hashimoto's we also need to address underlying gut infections. While that is the subject of my next book here are some tests to consider when you are ready to go this step.

- Biohealth 401 H
- CBC with inflammatory markers
- Cyrex Array #2
- Autonomic Response Testing
- Genova. www.gdx.net

Chapter Summary

- ✓ Trust your gut feeling
- ✓ We all have a psychobiome
- ✓ The Vagus Nerve is key to healing
- ✓ Depression and anxiety often disappear when we heal the gut
- ✓ Different diets for different people
- ✓ 5 Gut Types
- ✓ Phases of digestion

The Nourished Gut

What to eat? Isn't this the first question on any given day?

I hesitate to use the word "diet." It carries images of denial and restriction, and it means different things to different people. Think about Weight Watchers. To their credit, they have helped millions lose weight, but its focus is weight loss, not health. They are brilliant at branding and using the power of community to build alliances and loyalty, but this is not a diet that builds health.

Our focus with Hashimoto's is healing the gut. We eat to heal and nourish. As you take this journey, there are 5 stages most of my patients go through.

"What can I eat"

Stage 1 – Disbelief – "What? I can't eat pasta, cookies, granola anymore?"

Stage 2 – Resistance – "I know I should do it and I want to do it, but it's so hard. Maybe I'll try it a little bit."

Stage 3 – Agreement – "I agree that it would be beneficial for me to make these changes, so tell me how I can begin with a simple change."

Stage 4 – Acceptance – "I accept that my body is asking for help and that I can no longer do what I use to do and get a different result."

Stage 5 – Choice – "I choose to make these choices because I understand my 'why.' My 'why' is because I want to feel better, have more energy, get my creative juices back, feel strong enough to participate in life, and replenish and repair."

What makes this even more of a challenge is that two people with the exact same diagnosis may need very different diet strategies. This is because of our cultural influences, lifestyles, individual food sensitivities, and physiological response vary from one person to the next. Have you noticed that one diet works wonders for your friend, but for you it did nothing?

It can be very confusing to navigate the various options. I've provided a roadmap here. This is a guide, but just like reading a map, you sometimes have to consider there may be detours, toll roads, a scenic road, and the direct route.

You may find yourself moving from one to another as you move along your 'healing the gut' journey.

What makes this road even more challenging is there is not one diet that is right for everyone. Along with all the factors that influence diet choice, we also have 5 different Gut Types to consider.

In 1996, Dr. D'Adamo wrote the NY Times Bestseller *Eat Right For Your Type*. We learned that blood type antigens are prominent in our digestive tract, and because of this, many of the bacteria in your digestive tract actually use your blood type as a preferred food supply. Dr. D'Adamo created diets for each type, and many had great success just by eating for their blood type diets and lifestyle.

Now Dr. Josh Axe has combined contemporary physiology with traditional Chinese medicine, recognizied 5 Gut Types, and he illuminates for us what's unique to each type.

Stressed

A person with a "stressed" gut type often has issues around fear. Think of your childhood friend who would sometimes "pee their pants" when they became anxious or excited. These people may have underlying kidney/bladder/adrenal issues. They typically do better with blue and black foods like blueberries and kale.

Toxic

The "toxic" gut type may suffer from frustration or and/or anger. They often have difficulty digesting fats, and this may cause the small intestine to work harder to break down fats. Milk thistle, artichokes and arugula can be very helpful for this type

Immune

The "Immune" gut type may have increased irritable bowel syndrome and a lot of food sensitivities. They may suffer from grief or depression. Remember the vagus nerve we talked about that influences neurotransmitters that affect mood? The colon is often affected, and sometimes the GAPS (Gut And Psychology Syndrome) diet can be very helpful

Gastric

This type may suffer from acid reflux and often have sympathetic dominance with underlying emotional heart issues. Bitters can be helpful, along with fermented foods.

Candida

Dampness in the body affecting the stomach/spleen/pancreas is often found in this patient. They tend to be anxious and worrisome. They must avoid cold foods. They do well with cooked foods and warming stews.

Author of "*Hashimoto's: Finding the Root Cause,*" Dr. Izabella Wentz, collected information on 2,232 Hashimoto's patients. She compared the data of people who went on various types of diets and how it made them feel in terms of their symptoms, and what percentage of people had a reduction in antibodies as a result.

Food Survey Says...

Intervention	Felt Better	Felt Worse	Reduced Antibodies
Food Sensitivity	62%	4.20%	43%
AIP	75%	4%	38%
Soy Free	63%	1.20%	34%
Gluten Free	88%	0.73%	33%
Grain Free	81%	0.74%	28%
Paleo	81%	3.20%	27%
Low FODMAPs	39%	0%	27%

We can see that "gluten free" scored high for patients feeling better and reducing antibodies. Although identifying and removing the food sensitivities came in at 43% for reducing antibodies! Going grain free, Paleo, and Autoimmune Paleo (AIP) had very good results for many.

What is the food sensitivity diet?

We approach this diet with patients in three different ways.

In our office we offer muscle testing as taught by Dietrich Klinghardt, M.D., Ph.D, called Autonomic Response Testing. Klinghardt trained practitioners rely on this almost exclusively for identifying food sensitivities. The reason is it's the most reliable. Lab testing is not always accurate and again the same blood sample sent to the same lab may result in different findings.

Most people are surprised to learn that even "good" foods may not be the "right" foods. If you have access to a Klinghardt-trained practitioner, this is an excellent choice.

A simple start is to do a food elimination. The biggest culpri? many are: gluten, dairy, and sugar. After 30–90, days beg slowly reintroduce one at a time and keep a record of your symptoms, including bloating, brain fog, constipation, diarrhea, etc.

There is also blood testing for food sensitivity. Each practitioner seems to find their favorite labs, and I would recommend working with someone who has experience in testing and interpreting the results.

You can then take this information and apply it to the diet model you are following. Example: Paleo allows potatoes, but if you have a food sensitivity to potatoes, you would eliminate them.

A good place to begin is with the basic elimination diet (sugar, wheat, dairy), and then move toward a wider elimination.

Basic Elimination

Soy, dairy, corn, gluten, eggs, sugar, tree nuts

Most people will see benefits after a few weeks of eliminating these triggers and this can be a good place to begin.

Full Elimination may include

- Nightshades
- All Grains
- Nuts
- Personal allergies or sensitivities

Specialty Elimination

There can be sensitivities of varying degrees to certain compounds such as:

- Oxalates
- Glutamates
- Amines
- Salicylates

The following "diets" are designed to act as healthy medicine for the body. Typically, many do also lose weight on them, but this is not the objective. These diets are meant to be initiated for short periods with a focus on a particular goal or healing of symptoms. As you begin to heal, you may find that you will incorporate two or more of these diet solutions. Let's explore each of them for how they may be of value to you.

Autoimmune Paleo (AIP)

The autoimmune Paleo is for the patient who is dealing with autoimmune issues. This diet is more restrictive than the traditional Paleo program as it also excludes nuts, seeds, eggs, and legumes. Helpful for

- Healing leaky gut
- Decreasing autoimmune triggers
- Food allergies/sensitivities
- www.aiplifestyle.com

There are many books, classes, Facebook groups, and blogs available to learn more.

Gluten Free

This is a big topic and there are many perspectives. Some say it is a problem because of the genetic hybridization (GMO), others because of the glyphosate (active ingredient in Round-Up), and others say it is the antibodies that are produced in response to gluten.

In part this is because there are good glutens and bad glutens. Bad gluten is found in wheat, rye, oats, and barley. But gluten can also be found in quinoa, rice, and other grains. Some people can digest rice proteins but may not be able to digest wheat gluten. There are gluten containing compounds in everything from barbecue sauce to bouillon and chewing gum to condiments.

Part of the problem is that most people will say, "I eat wheat and I feel fine." When you have a gluten intolerance there is a delayed reaction. The reaction gradually builds over time, and with continued exposure it's harder for us to make the correlation between what we ate and how we feel. The testing is not very specific, which leads to many false negatives and false positives, so the gold standard for gluten sensitivity is still by elimination.

There is a wealth of information available on how to live a gluten-free lifestyle, and this is the first step we have our Hashimoto's patients take.

Recommended reading: *No Grain, No Pain* by Dr. Peter Osborne

Paleo

Grains, legumes, dairy, and sugar are all eliminated, with an emphasis placed on grass-fed, wild caught, pasture-raised, organic, and locally grown food, and good, healthy fats.

Very helpful for:

- Weight loss
- Inflammation
- Stabilize blood sugar
- Autoimmune disorders
- Improve digestion
- Fibromyalgia and pain syndromes

Low FODMAP'S diet

Fermentable Oligo-Di-Monosaccharides and Polyols.

This may be a good choice for those with digestive issues such as IBS or Crohn's, Celiac.

It is based on the chemical structure of certain foods, including monosaccharides, disaccharides, and polysaccharides. Only monosaccharides are allowed on the diet as they are more easily absorbed. By limiting the complex carbs, the bad bacteria are not being fed.

Does not include grains, but for those patients that can tolerate them, nuts, dairy, and eggs are included.

Recommendation:

Breaking the Vicious Cycle by Elaine Gottschall

Other popular and effective programs:

Gut & Psychology Syndrome (GAPS)

GAPS was created by Dr. Natasha Campbell McBride

It has its roots in the SCD diet, but refined for patients who deal with intestinal/neurological issues.

Indicated for

- Learning disabilities
- Autism
- Depression
- ADHD
- Psychiatric disorders
- Digestive Disorders
- Food Allergies/sensitivities

Focuses on removing foods that are difficult to digest and that damage the gut flora. An emphasis is placed on fermented food and healing broths.

May not be helpful for someone who has had their gallbladder removed or issues with digesting fats.

Recommended: www.gapsdiet.com

Ketogenic

This diet was originally created to help treat patients with epilepsy by providing a high fat, adequate protein, low-carb diet. Regaining popularity many are embracing it for high performance sports, weight loss and chronic Lyme Disease.

A large focus is on the specific combination of foods and how the body metabolizes them for increased energy. Fat is converted in the liver into fatty acids and ketones. With time, the body turns from burning glucose for energy to burning fat for energy.

Helpful In

- Brain injuries
- Parkinson's disease
- Epilepsy
- ADHD
- Depression
- Blood sugar regulation

www.ketogenic-diet-resource.com

Body Ecology

Focus is on the "inner ecology" of the body. Specific attention on food combination using whole foods, food combining, good fats, and cultured foods. Yeast such as candida produce acetaldehyde, a very toxic chemical. If the body is chronically exposed to this chemical, it can accumulate in body tissues and prevent T3 getting into the cells as well as restrict T4 from converting to T3. Alcoholics have large amount of this toxicity in their liver. Clearing out our liver allows for better conversion of hormones, which lead to the remission of Hashimoto's. Acetaldehyde can be harmful to the adrenals as well.

Eliminating sugar is the first step.

If candida is a problem, the Body Ecology diet can be tremendously helpful.

Antibody or stool testing can be helpful for identifying candida.

Helpful for

- Candida overgrowth
- Severe digestive distress
- Gut dysbiosis
- ADD/ADHD related to imbalanced flora

Recommended: www.bodyecology.com

NOTE: If you find you are reacting to fermented foods you may want to be evaluated for SIBO. Small intestinal bacterial overgrowth has been found in about 50% of patients with thyroid disorders.You can start off with the Bifidus family of probiotics, which do not produce the lactic acid.

Recommendation:

Flora Baby available from RenewLife.

If you have done gene testing like 23 and Me and you have the FUT 2 gene, then you may be prone to B12 issues and keeping bifidus in the gut. Diversity is the secret to a healthy gut. Diversity is the secret to humanity.

Microbiome Diet

Created by Raphael Kellman, MD, to help restore the microbiome and influence weight loss, gastrointestinal health, depression, anxiety, and insomnia.

Incorporates superfoods, fermented foods, natural probiotics, and prebiotics.

Recommended: *The Microbiome Diet* by Raphael Kellman, MD.

The reasons we always begin patient care by addressing the gut are two-fold. Number 1: More than 80 million Americans suffer from digestive issues. Number 2: By addressing the gut and rebalancing and repairing, you are also impacting detoxification pathways, supporting the liver, and allowing the body to reduce inflammation. This frees up energy for the body to work on other long-needed repairs.

While diet is a critical component of reducing the inflammation in Hashimoto's and healing the gut, the solution for complete remission must also address adrenals, toxins, methylation issues, pathogens, and infections, as well as unhealed emotional trauma.

Bonus tip: Coca Pulse Test

Relax for about five minutes. Measure your pulse. Eat one food you may be curious about as to whether you have a sensitivity. Eat the food. Relax for fifteen minutes.

Take your pulse again; if it has increased 15 or more beats there is a high certainty. Increased by 10–14 beats, a possible allergy.

Chapter Summary

✓ What to eat is different for every person

✓ Identify your food sensitivities and triggers

✓ Begin with an elimination diet

✓ Good food is not always the right food

✓ 5 Stages of "What can I eat?"

5 R's: Remove, Replenish, Repair, Re-inoculate, Rebalance

This step can be very frustrating for patients because it takes time. We often have to spend quite a bit of time helping patients understand each step so they can become their own advocates. Chronic disease began in the body long before it was detected. Rebalancing the body also takes time and there is a natural progression.

Each of these steps is vital and is based on individual history, symptoms, and need. Working with a Functional Medicine Practitioner or holistic and integrated coach will help you prioritize and guide you through the steps.

This is a sequence we guide each patient through on their journey to healing. Each step is interdependent and they all build upon the other.

Remove

Imagine you want to paint your kitchen and bathroom. You have been living there for over 10 years and have accumulated many appliances, dishes, and towels, and the cabinets and counters are brimming with everyday tools.

Before you can paint you have to first REMOVE the objects and items that are in your way. In some cases, you may even have to sand, prime, or prepare the walls for the new color.

This is exactly the same with the body. Too often, we see many patients who followed a detox or cleanse on the internet without preparing the drainage pathways and organs of elimination. They may find themselves feeling worse than they did before they began the program.

When we think about "remove," these are some of the things we consider:

Identify and remove the triggers – Sometimes we do not even know what the triggers are, especially with food intolerance, where we may have a delayed reaction or no symptom at all.

Food sensitivities (gluten, soy, dairy, sugar) 30-day elimination diet. Alcohol and foods containing capsaicin such as peppers.

Toxins

This list is growing every day. With ongoing exposure to everyday cleaners, chemtrails, pesticides, herbicides, air fresheners, and more, we are constantly bombarded by chemicals that are disrupting our pathways and competing for receptor sites for necessary molecules like hormones and neurotransmitters.

Infections

No matter how good a diet you are eating, if there are parasites and other intestinal infections, you will need more than food to address these pathogens.

Parasites

Patients are quite surprised when we even mention the word. They are under the false impression that parasites are only found in Third World countries. Not so. As the global world has become smaller and we are able to move freely around the globe we are exposed in one area and bringing it to the next place we travel to.

Emotional triggers

Food and emotions are topics that many great books have been written about. Growing up in an Italian family, my inner picture of family is that we gather on Sunday around a big family table and enjoy pasta and wine and all the smells and sights that go along with it. Sometimes the feeling is so strong that my husband and I will just have to have a traditional Sunday Sauce kind of day, and then our emotional heart is satisfied.

We all have these triggers. For fun, I asked my Facebook community, as our region was preparing for a 3-day snow-in, what foods they were already planning on making. The answers ranged from a pot of stew and soup to peanut butter and banana on white bread sandwiches. Some wanted hot dogs and others wanted hot chocolate and cookies. We all have memories from our childhood – some conscious and some unconscious – of snow days as a child, and we crave that comfort. These are our emotional triggers around food. It's common, and we must prepare for them and have alternatives in place to avoid a complete meltdown.

Behaviors

If your typical behavior is stopping at the local Dunkin Donuts or having drinks after work every day, you will have to re-think these behaviors and make appropriate changes.

Negative Thinking

Whether it's your "stinkin' thinkin'" or someone you encounter, you can bet that not everyone will agree with your decision to make these changes.

One of my biggest pet peeves is when I visit a seriously ill person in the hospital, and they bring in their food tray laced with things like chlorinated and fluoridated water, overcooked pesticide-ridden vegetables, and sweeteners like Splenda and bleached sugar. Hormone-induced, toxic, pesticide-injected milk that does nothing to help these patients are some of the biggest offenders. Yet, we never even ask the question, "Is this good for me?" We want to believe that someone has actually given this some thought and is protecting us. Sorry, folks. Hospitals are corporations, and they are in business to serve their shareholders. They do that by getting you in and out as fast as they can with as little cost and as little risk to them as possible.

I recently found myself sitting in a salon next to a female OB-Gyn, and we struck up a conversation. I asked her opinion as to why she thought the increase of Caesareans has been so ongoing. She told me that doctors make the same fee whether the baby is vaginal birth or Caesarean, but the big difference has to do with insurance malpractice. Doctors are protected by their malpractice if the baby is born by C-section and there's a problem, but less protected by a compromised delivery through the vaginal canal. This is pure nonsense.

Chemicals

One of the things I like to do is a search on the active ingredients in products. Cleaning products, personal products, household products, and more. I am sad to say that often the very ingredient that we rely on to do the work is not only a known carcinogen, but it is often banned in every other country except the USA.

Start learning how to use natural cleaners like baking soda, white vinegar, borax, and essential oils. I can now clean my house from top to bottom with only these ingredients, without harming the environment or my family.

Electromagnetic Sensitivity

This is a condition of the new millennium. Wi-fi, cordless phones, cell phones, cell towers, and baby monitors, along with smart chips and smart meters, carry an electromagnetic field that is turning out to be quite dangerous for some. While everyone is impacted, the degree to which you will be affected is dependent on many factors.

Sleep in a device-free, EMF-free bedroom. This should be your sanctuary. Sleep is when our bodies move into a parasympathetic state to begin the repair work of the day. When the body is not able to access this state, we end up with a central nervous system disorder and/or neuralgias, paresthesias, numbness, and tingling that strains our bodies and leaves us feeling confused and numbed.

MOLD

Environmental toxins – Every home and workplace needs to be evaluated for sick building syndrome, leaks, mold, or other toxins that prevent us from healing and feeling whole.

I personally left a dream home that had become a "sick house." This puts enormous stress on families, as one member may be highly reactive and the other members are not. This is a serious issue and must be considered in anyone healing from an autoimmune disease. You cannot get well in a sick house.

Replenish

After a workout, long day at the office or even a day in the garden requires us to take time to "replenish"... hydrate, rest, nourish and give back vital nutrients to revitalize our body.

Think of the body as hardware and software. The physical body is the hardware and the internal microbiome is the software. They communicate by electrical, chemical, and light messengers.

Enzymes & Bitters

The number one cause of internal toxicity is undigested food resulting from an enzyme-depleted diet. For us to thrive, we must be able to efficiently digest and absorb nutrients and eliminate waste products efficiently. When you have gut issues, this is one of the foundational tools we use.

Historically, enzymes required for digestion were obtained from our food. However, due to the nutrient-poor soil, genetic engineering, processing pesticide use, and chemical fertilizers, these enzymes have been depleted and often require replacement.

It is estimated that between 60% and 70% of our energy goes towards digestion. An enzyme-depleted diet requires a greater input of pancreatic enzymes for digestion.

It's helpful to do some pre-testing to know if you have acid, enzyme, or other production deficiencies. If you have had your gallbladder removed, then enzymes are essential.

Seek out products without binders and fillers. Fillers can be: starch, calcium salts and sugars, like lactose. Binders are added to create compression such as: starch, cellulose or sucrose.

Natural ways to increase enzymes in your diet:

- Increase the amount of raw food in your diet. Sprouts contain 30–35% protein, lots of enzymes, and you can grow your own.
- Chew, chew, chew. Chewing mixes the food with your salivary enzymes and improves the digestion of your food.
- Teaspoon of organic apple cider vinegar 15 minutes before a meal.
- Eat ginger. Ginger increases the activity of lipase and other digestive enzymes that stimulate bile flow.
- Eat more fermented foods.

- Bitters. Bitters have been used for millennia to stimulate and improve digestion. Use them just before a meal. There are many products on the market. Look for high-quality ingredients or learn to make your own. One of my favorite formulas combines dandelion, milk thistle, gentian, burdock, and essential oils of orange, myrrh, juniper, and clove.

How to use enzymes with HCL

Adequate levels of HCL are necessary for absorption of protein, calcium, vitamin B12, and more. Hydrochloric acid serves many functions, including being a protective barrier and killing many potentially harmful micro-organisms.

Many people with Hashimoto's have low stomach acid, which leads to improper digestion of foods, which leads to deficiencies and more food sensitivities and more fatigue.

Betaine with pepsin is recommended, but everyone has to find the dosage that is correct for them. Begin with 1 capsule after a protein-rich meal. If you did not experience any burning in the throat or stomach, at the next meal increase to 2 and then 3 accordingly. Example: If you took 4 capsules and experienced discomfort, then back down to 3 capsules.

pH

Did you ever care for a fish tank or swimming pool, checking the pH to insure the water was the proper pH to allow for safe swimming and an algae-free environment? It is no different in the body. We can test the pH in the saliva and the urine and we expect them to be different. The pH of the body controls and affects all the functions of the body. A diet high in acid-producing foods and/or chronic stress can disrupt the acid/base balance. In order to re-establish balance, the body will use its essential mineral stores to buffer the acidic environment. When the pH in the gut is too acidic, it allows for parasites and other unfriendly organisms to take up room in our bodies. When it comes to the body ecology, it is all about creating a balance, or homeostasis, so that we encourage symbiotic relationships and commensal harmony among the microbes. By recording your pH over 5 days and taking the average, you can estimate the acidity in your body and make the corrections as necessary. Eating a more alkaline diet, which is a diet higher in plants, and increasing your water absorption can help a great deal.

Measure your urine 5 days in a row using Hydrion pH paper. Dismiss the high and low, then average the middle three. Ideal first morning urinary pH is 6.4–7.0.

How can your body get too acidic?

- Excessive intake of acid-producing foods and decreased intake of alkalizing foods
- Excess stress
- Inflammation
- Imbalance in intestinal flora
- Lack of optimal exercise
- Lack of fresh air
- Medications

How to balance your body pH value:

- Make dietary adjustments, balancing acid and alkaline foods
- Optimize fluid intake
- Optimize exercise
- Manage stress levels

Colon health

Assess your bowel movements. How often are you going? What is the transit time? What is the consistency, shape of your stools, consider the odor and the color. A daily bowel movement does not necessarily indicate a healthy colon. Even if you are having a daily bowel movement, are you eliminating the last meal or a meal you enjoyed three days ago? The only way to know is to do a bowel transit test. Bowel transit time is the amount of time it takes for foot to travel through the digestive tract. The ideal bowel transit time is between 12 and 24 hours. A transit time of greater than 2 days can increase the risk of cancer, diverticulosis, and candidiasis.

Test your bowel transit time by taking activated charcoal and notice how long before your stools turn dark, or eat a cup of beets and count the number of hours before you see you see a change in your stool.

We strive to have stools shaped like type #4.

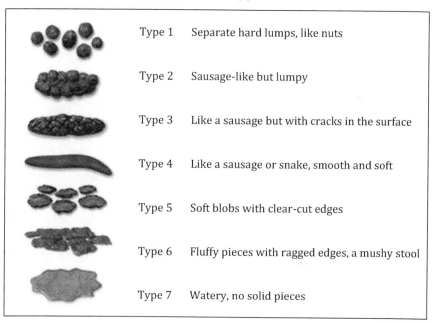

	Type 1	Separate hard lumps, like nuts
	Type 2	Sausage-like but lumpy
	Type 3	Like a sausage but with cracks in the surface
	Type 4	Like a sausage or snake, smooth and soft
	Type 5	Soft blobs with clear-cut edges
	Type 6	Fluffy pieces with ragged edges, a mushy stool
	Type 7	Watery, no solid pieces

Hydration

Water makes up more than 70% of the body's tissues and plays a role in nearly every body function, from regulating temperature and cushioning joints to bringing oxygen to the cells and removing waste from the body. How much water do you need? To function as an optimal level we suggest one quart for every 50 lbs of body weight.

Not all water is the same. This IS A BIG deal. The best form of water is spring water from a tested source. You can improve the quality of drinking water by filtering with a reverse osmosis system, charcoal, ceramic, or gravity filter. Store water in glass and avoid PVC or clear plastic water bottles you find at the store. We encourage patients to restructure their water as well.

Cellular Communication

Think of it this way. Our cells are dynamic energetic units. The liver needs to know what the gallbladder is thinking and the heart needs to know what the brain knows. They have a unique fiberoptic-like communication system that is dependent on trace minerals and electrolytes and light input. The processing of foods and deficient soils has led to a severe mineral deficiency for most of the population.

Ensure your health program provides for these vital components.

Repair

We are not what we eat, but we are what we assimilate, absorb, and excrete.

Hydrochloric Acid

Once food makes its way to the stomach, it is the hydrochloric acid that helps to not only break the food down, but also plays a protective role against harmful bacteria and pathogens. As we grow older our levels of HCL begin to decline. HCL also triggers the release of enzymes like pepsin needed for digestion, as well as alkaline bicarbonate into the blood.

Undigested food ferments in the gut and putrifies. This breakdown produces unhealthy levels of the gas ammonia which begins to leak into the bloodstream, resulting in symptoms such as: fatigue, skin rashes, anxiety, and more.

The mucous membranes of our gut act as a barrier from HCL reaching to areas other than the stomach. We begin to see that everything impacts something else.

Ayurvedic practitioners have long understood the benefits of consuming celery juice to build HCL. In addition to being a good source of Vitamin K, C, potassium, folate, and fiber, it contains a beneficial sodium complex that is useful in raising our hydrochloric acid.

Methylation pathways

One of these important pathways is Methylation. This is what occurs when the body takes one substance and turns it into another so it is detoxified and excreted. In this case, a carbon atom with 3 hydrogen atoms (a methyl group) attaches to another molecule, turning one molecule into another that fosters detoxification. This process is essential for the proper function of almost all of your body's systems. It occurs billions of times every second; it helps repair your DNA on a daily basis, it controls homocysteine (an unhealthy compound that can damage blood vessels), it helps recycle molecules needed for detoxification, and it helps maintain mood and keep inflammation in check.

Nearly everyone with autoimmune thyroid disease has problems with their genes from methylation. A useful test is knowing your homocysteine levels. If your homocysteine is below ten, your body is doing a decent job with methylation reactions. This is a good gauge of how the function of methylation is being carried out.

Toxins slow down the methylation process by stealing methyl groups, and infections like *h.Pylori* deplete the B-vitamins, minerals, Vitamin D, and gut flora.

If you are struggling with health and not improving, it may be helpful to understand your methylation pathways in order to optimize health. Be sure you are getting Riboflavin (B2) Methylfolate, and B12. Restrict use of folic acid or synthetic folic acid. Go to MTHFR.net and watch videos and read articles.

Recommendations: Homocysteine Factor is helpful for people with the MTHFR gene mutation. Homocysteine Supreme from Designs for Health is also beneficial. They have the the activated B6 and activated methylfolate and methylcobalamin. Take 2 capsules per day. Also, continue to monitor your homocysteine levels.

Testing:

www.23andme.com

www.Geneticgenie.com

Repair the gut wall by addressing the mucous membranes of the gut

This system is protected by a certain tissue known as GALT. GALT is an acronym for Gut Associated Lymphoid Tissue, and more than 60% of the immune function of the body is contained in GALT. This GALT is part of our immune response that forms our defensive army of T & B lymphocytes that are responsible for carrying out attacks and producing antibodies against antigens or anything the body thinks is an invader.

Constant assault on the digestive system by acidic foods, bacteria, viruses, or other irritants can result in damage to this delicate lining of the small intestine. This damage impairs the digestive process, leading to poor absorption of nutrients and putrefaction of undigested food particles. Just as tonsils carry immune cells and immune proteins, the GALT protects the bloodstream from anything that might find its way through the the gut and into the bloodstream.

In response to this constant assault, cells in the small intestine release a layer of protective mucus, seeking to lubricate and protect themselves from further damage. In his book *Grain Brain*, Dr. Pearlmutter says a similar problem can happen in the brain. The blood-brain barrier is designed like the GALT tissue to protect the brain from things like bacterial microbes and damaging chemicals. Some of the very same mechanisms that give leaky gut can create leaky brain. Leaky gut = leaky brain.

Recommendations:

- L-Glutamine – Helps repair intestinal lining
- N-Acetyl Cysteine – Helps restore gut lining, antioxidant, liver function, helps eliminate pathogenic bacteria – 1800 mg daily with food
- Aloe Vera – soothing and anti-inflammatory
- Curcumin – Anti-inflammatory
- Omega 3's
- Cod Liver Oil
- Zinc – Required for T4 to T3 conversion
- Butyrate – ghee and butter are excellent sources
- Colostrum

Herbs to consider:

- Slippery Elm
- Marshmallow

Re-inoculate

Imagine you are in charge of seeding a new planet. Your job is to ensure a wide variety of soil-rich organisms with multiple responsibilities to provide the nourishment for your people. This is simple, but it is not easy. Our inner ecosystem is a dynamic system and it is constantly changing.

Therefore we need a variety of beneficial microflora or "friendly" bacteria living in our gut. There is no one pre- or probiotic that will provide us with all that is required.

You can choose powdered, capsules, or liquid probiotics.

Recommendations:

- http://restore4life.com/
- Soil based organisms – www.prescriptassist.com
- VSL#3

- Ther-biotic by Klaire Labs

Begin to shift your mindset on how you think of bacteria. In the right composition and balance, they are truly our friends.

Shift away from products like hand sanitizers. Let your hands get dirty. Walk barefoot, once again exposing yourself to billions of organisms.

Fermented Foods

Fermented foods are an ancient tradition of providing people with a rich biodiversity of living, healthy bacteria. You can learn to make your own or find them in the refrigerated section of your favorite health food store. Each batch will differ, even with the same recipe. We have found it best to do some of the earlier work first before adding fermented foods.

Think of it this way. You recently moved into a new neighborhood and you would like to meet your neighbors. You could start off with a block party with loud music and lots of food, or you may choose to bring a box of cookies to your nearest neighbor. They both may work, but the big party may be a bit more invasive for some. When you introduce new bacteria the whole "guild" will respond appropriately. To alleviate a reaction of gas and bloating, it is best to start small and go slow.

Resistant Starch

Resistant starch is a different approach, as it is providing food for the probiotic bacteria. What's interesting about this is that resistant starch travels through the gastrointestinal tract without being broken down and becoming fuel for the cells. Instead, this becomes fuel for the bacteria in the colon, where it is converted to short-chain fatty acids, one of which is called butyrate. Butyrate not only helps the colon to rebuild, repair, and replenish, but it helps to lower cancer risk and increase the population of good

colon bacteria to ward off disease. Butyrate is like a su
your colon, and resistant starch is how you deliver that

Foods that contain resistant starch include:

- Cooked and cooled potatoes (potato flour and /or starch)
- Green bananas
- Green plantains
- Legumes such as lentils and chickpeas
- Cashews
- Raw oats

Butyrate also improves insulin sensitivity and increases the amount of fat that is burned as energy. The highest concentration of butyrate may be found in high-quality grass-fed butter. When we eat foods high in fiber and resistant starch, our bacteria feed on it and produce butyric acid from it. Jerusalem artichokes, jicama, leeks, asparagus, and onions are fibrous foods to fill up on.

Rebalance

Change is often uncomfortable for many. Motivational speaker and author, Anthony Robbins, often says you won't change until the issue you are trying to move away from becomes more painful than the pain you imagine of having to change.

We are creatures of habit, familiarity, and comfort. Change is uncomfortable. It's especially difficult if you are wanting to change your diet and your husband and children are not on board. My husband is blessed with a gut like a goat! Basically, he seems to eat whatever he wants and never has any discomfort. It's quite remarkable to watch him eat hot dogs and cheese sandwiches while washing it down with his favorite beer. My husband rarely misses a day of work because he is sick, and if he does get sick, he rebounds within 48 hours. He has a wonderful constitution. I came to learn that he grew up on fermented foods, and to this day, he enjoys not only fermented foods, but growing his own sprouts. I would have to conclude his microbiome is so strong that he has been able to adapt and respond to whatever environment he finds himself in. He has excellent methylation and detoxification pathways. He absorbs, excretes, and assimilates with ease.

Not so for me or most of the patients we encounter. It is a daily balancing act of self care blended with whole foods and mindfulness. It requires time, commitment, and desire. You must desire to change. Your 'why' needs to be bigger than your 'why not.'

My 'why' is two-fold. Number one, I would not make a good patient. I move at a brisk pace and am quite active. I did my first triathlon at age 60 just to challenge myself. I have 5 grandchildren ranging in age from 2–13, and I plan on dancing at their weddings. Therefore, I must take action today to protect and rebalance my health.

We all know friends and family who lived well and may have died quite young anyway, from some disease or trauma. We do not know the future. Taking good care of yourself is a form of insurance, but it is not a guarantee that you will not get sick. However, I have seen when people have lived a good life, they tend to not only recover more quickly, but their end days lean toward a higher quality of life. They drive longer, remain mobile, and are still quick-witted. Aging is not an option, but how we age is completely within our choices.

Lifestyle changes

I remind you we are social organisms. We have an innate instinct to bond and gather. Social genomics are showing us that those who enjoy community and relationships not only age better, but live longer healthfully. When you are ready to make lifestyle changes, seek out others who have similar goals. Support each other. Find a buddy. Join a walking club or a garden club or whatever group that aligns with your personal health goals. You will find renewed strength, courage, desire, and momentum.

Behavior modifications

We each have our own style for this type of change. When my husband decided to stop smoking 35 years ago, he put them down on New Year's Eve and said he would never smoke again. He didn't. Others need a different approach. Maybe make smaller changes one at a time. It doesn't matter how you approach it, just as long as you do. Find your style and stick with it. You'll get there!

Eating patterns

Chew, chew, chew. Sadly, our restaurants do not encourage quiet and tranquil atmospheres for ease of digestion. In fact, it's quite opposite. Today, you go into a restaurant and your attention is diverted to blaring TV screens, each with a different event, and music loudly blaring from the speakers, all with a backdrop of tables set too close to the others and loud conversations competing for your attention.

Our parasympathetic nervous system needs to be engaged and activated for easy digestion. This system cannot be accessed when we find ourself in this competing environment. Make a conscious choice to set a lovely table, speak a prayer of thanks over your food, and chew, chew, chew. Chewing stimulates the digestive enzymes naturally secreted by the body that are required to break down the food into the nutrients and compounds that will nourish and repair.

Emotional needs

When you have a desire to binge or eat badly, take a breath and ask yourself, "What am I feeling?" Are you experiencing loneliness, anger, boredom, or some other feeling that is needing your attention? We often use food to suppress other feelings, and when we can get in touch with the feeling we can move away from the table and into our heart.

Exercise program

We are designed to move. We live in a culture that keeps us sitting at a desk all day and on a couch at night. We can navigate our lives with a remote, a smart phone, and a laptop. These tools have brought great opportunity into our lives, but they come with a cost.

Moving is now something that we have to choose, for most of us are not making our living as farmers or construction workers or athletes. We have to choose to move. Start with small steps. Increase a little each day. Soon you will find yourself feeling more limber and flexible and stronger. Your body will thank you, and the satisfaction of fitting into your favorite jeans and the reflection in the mirror will make you smile.

Spiritual journey

This is not religion. There is a difference. A spiritual tone is one that recognizes the beauty and connection of nature and our relationship to all things. When we live from a place of building bridges and community instead of walls and separation, we find a deep peace that resonates in every action and encounter. This peace cannot be bought, but it can be cultivated just like a healthy gut.

Chapter Summary

- ✓ Remove – Triggers, obstacles, behaviors that know longer serve you
- ✓ Digital Detox weekly
- ✓ Create a Sleep Sanctuary
- ✓ Check for mold
- ✓ Replenish enzymes, pH, colon health and hydration
- ✓ Repair – the gut wall and detoxification pathways

✓ Re-inoculate- Explore fermented foods and resistant starch

✓ Rebalance – Explore your feelings around change, start an exercise program, consider your spiritual journey

Gut Solutions

Your Aha!

Part of my desire to write this book was to help you understand your "why." As a practitioner I have learned that if a patient is not motivated to change, they probably will not. I hope you have found your why in the pages of this little book. We have talked about the "what" and "why," and now we want to address the "how."

The "how" is going to be different for each of us. While the most important step is to "remove" the triggers and follow along the 5 R's, the how depends on a lot of factors. Budget, time, culture, food sensitivities, belief systems, and willingness. Those patients who are willing to put in the time and make the appropriate changes often see very positive and rewarding results in a relatively short time. Once you begin to have the energy and return to your "normal" healthy and happy self you will be inspired to continue.

Being a practitioner has provided me with a front row seat to the health challenges and healing journeys of many. I clearly see that health is NOT a one-size-fits-all approach. In fact, it is very individual. Perhaps, as individual as the microbiome that is uniquely yours. Below are some of the top strategies which have helped many. Give them a chance to work for you. You'll be glad you did.

As I began to gather my notes from my years of practice, what got my attention is how many of the treatments that work best are some of the oldest practices people have known and embraced. It's also clear that what changed was our thinking. We began to move away from natural practices and were swept away by the hype and marketing of newer technology, more bells and whistles, and the changing landscape of how doctors "doctor".

Takeaways

We have moved away from what the idea of real food is. REAL FOOD DOES NOT COME IN A BOX.

GERMS ARE NOT THE ENEMY.

Factors That Affect Thyroid Function

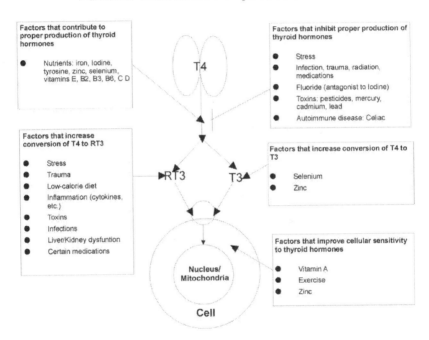

Factors that contribute to proper production of thyroid hormones

- Nutrients: iron, Iodine, tyrosine, zinc, selenium, vitamins E, B2, B3, B6, C D

Factors that increase conversion of T4 to RT3

- Stress
- Trauma
- Low-calorie diet
- Inflammation (cytokines, etc.)
- Toxins
- Infections
- Liver/Kidney dysfuntion
- Certain medications

Factors that inhibit proper production of thyroid hormones

- Stress
- Infection, trauma, radiation, medications
- Fluoride (antagonist to Iodine)
- Toxins: pesticides, mercury, cadmium, lead
- Autoimmune disease: Celiac

Factors that increase conversion of T4 to T3

- Selenium
- Zinc

Factors that improve cellular sensitivity to thyroid hormones

- Vitamin A
- Exercise
- Zinc

T4

RT3   T3

Nucleus/ Mitochondria

Cell

Even good foods may not be the Right foods – Learn to Test

Muscle testing comes in many forms, from Applied Kinesiology to Autonomic Response Testing and Nutritional Response Testing to O-ring. There is a science and an art in all muscle testing.

No matter which technique you are drawn to, we recommend all our patients learn to muscle test for their personal and family benefit.

With the chronic disease states we find in patients, one of the best treatments has been being able to customize treatment for each patient. Whether it is food, pathogens, toxins, or remedies we are testing, they affect each person as uniquely as their microbiome. Often remedies, supplements, foods, and tinctures must be "pulsed" and "rotated." This simply means pulsing the dose up and down and then rotating how the substance is taken.

Having the benefit of home muscle testing, you will be able to customize your treatments to you. You may test poorly for a food or remedy this week, but that may change in the future. Being able to monitor this with some reliable and consistent muscle testing will go a long way to your success in health and healing.

Vagus nerve Support

We talked about the Vagus nerve being a bidirectional highway for signaling between the gut and the brain. Reestablishing communication is essential in rebuilding this essential pathway. Experts recommend:

1. **Slow, rhythmic, diaphragmatic breathing.** Belly breathing from the diaphragm, not from the top of the lungs, stimulates and tones the vagus nerve.
2. **Humming.** Since the vagus nerve is connected to the vocal cords, humming mechanically stimulates it. You can hum a song, or even better, repeat the sound 'OM.'
3. **Speaking.** Making exaggerated vowel sounds for vagal tone, due to the connection to the vocal cords.
4. **Washing your face with cold water.** Diving Reflex; cold water on your face stimulates the vagus nerve.
5. **Meditation, especially loving-kindness meditation.** Heart-centered meditation promotes feelings of goodwill towards yourself and others. A 2010 study by Barbara Fredrickson and Bethany Kik found that increasing positive emotions led to increased social closeness, and an improvement in vagal tone.

6. ***Balancing the gut microbiome***. The presence of healthy bacteria in the gut creates a positive feedback loop through the vagus nerve, increasing its tone.

Gargling

Functional neurologist Datis Kharrazian, M.D., recommends activating the vagus nerve by gargling. It also stimulates the gut-brain axis. Simply pour 2 ounces of filtered water into a glass and gargle for as long as you can. Try and do it 2–3 times per day.

Balance your blood sugar

Balancing Blood Sugar Rules – Thanks to Dr. Isabella Wentz

1. Include fat/protein with every meal: eggs, nuts, seeds, fish, meat
2. Eat every two to three hours at first. Snacks are great!
3. No sweets before bed.
4. Avoid fruit juice.
5. Limit caffeine.
6. Avoid all grains and dairy, soy, corn, and yeast.
7. Eat breakfast within one hour of waking.
8. Include snacks rich in protein/fat every two to three hours.
9. No fasting.
10. Cut out foods with a glycemic index above 55.
11. Never skip breakfast.
12. Always combine carbohydrates with fat or protein.
13. Never exceed a 2:1 ratio of carb to protein.

Recommendation:

Berberine – A naturally occurring Alkaloid helpful for insulin resistance, balancing blood sugar, and increasing good bacteria. 500mg before each meal.

Chromium – Required nutrient for thyroid function and helpful with blood sugar regulation. 200–00 mcg

Niacin – 1,000 mg 2/day

Ketogenic Diet can be helpful

Eliminate refined carbohydrates. Limit potatoes and try to focus on foods that fall into a glycemic index below 55. Most non-starchy vegetables fall into this category. Reference www.glycemicindex.com for more information

Nutrient Deficiencies

We use a functional medicine interpretation of our patient's Complete Blood Chemistries (CBC). Most traditionally-trained medical practitioners only look for ranges outside the accepted values. To recognize nutrient deficiencies you need an understanding of the patterns, ratios, and trends the numbers are reflecting.

For example: This is a pattern we may see with a patient who has a need for B12/Folate: MCV ↑, LDH ↑, Albumin ↓, Total WBCs ↓, RBC, Female ↓, Hemoglobin, Female ↓, Hematocrit, Female ↓

A pattern to recognize a need for Vitamin C: Albumin ↓, Alk Phos ↑, RBC, Female ↓, Hemoglobin, Female ↓, Hematocrit, Female ↓, MCV ↑

You can clearly see there is more to understanding lab work than just the values that may fall outside the accepted range.

A functional medicine practitioner can be very helpful here. Some practitioners use Spectracell testing, which can be quite helpful. www.spectracell.com

You can read more about interpretation here: http://rasahealth.com/functional-blood-chemistry-analysis/

Vitamin D – Immune support, reduce inflammation, and autoimmune symptoms. Look for a formulation with K2 in a liposomal form. 5,000–10,000 IU

der Liposomal:

One of the drawbacks when taking supplements is malabsorption due to a compromised gut. We find many patients taking a lot of supplements that are not being utilized. Liposomal is a way of delivering the nutrient encased in a lipid case that facilitates absorption directly in the mouth or by preventing breakdown by the stomach acid. As the research of this form of delivery gains greater awareness and the technology becomes more available, you will begin to hear more about the benefits.

The other problem we see in many of the products our patients bring in is the amount of binders, flow agents, fillers, and toxic added ingredients. Even good products found in reliable health food stores have been found to include these. Learn to read the label and understand what you are reading.

Here is a list of ingredients best avoided in your supplements:

Colors

While FDA approved, Pfizer-owned brand supplements marketed as Centrum,contain toxic coloring agents like FD&C Blue No. 2 Aluminum Lake and FD&C Red No. 40 Aluminum Lake, both of which are potential neurotoxins. Even children's vitamins like Flintstones Complete contain these and other toxic coloring agents. (http://www.greenmedinfo.com)

Titanium Dioxide

Made from titanium bits, titanium dioxide has been linked to causing autoimmune disorders, cancer, and various other diseases. Besides the fact that it belongs to a class of particles known to cause cell damage, titanium dioxide serves no therapeutic purpose whatsoever, which means it does not belong in a health supplement.

"Titanium dioxide has recently been classified by the International Agency for Research on Cancer (IARC) as an IARC Group 2B carcinogen 'possibly carcinogen[ic] to humans,'" explains the Canadian Centre for Occupational Health & Safety on its website.

"This evidence showed that high concentrations of pigment-grade (powdered) and ultrafine titanium dioxide dust caused respiratory tract cancer in rats exposed by inhalation and intratracheal instillation."
(http://www.naturalnews.com/027000_titanium_dioxide_vitamins.html)

Supplements may contain flowing agents (talc), lubricants (magnesium stearate, calcium stearate, ascorbyl palmitate, hydrogenated vegetable oil) and binders such as dextrose sugar, polyethylene glycol and wax.

Supplements should be free of artificial additives, gluten, dairy, and soy.

Methylated forms of B12 (methylcobalamin) are better than cyanocobalamin

Folic Acid is best in the form of methylfolate

Capsules are generally better formulated than tablets but they may also contain added sugars and lubricants. Commercial products found at the drugstore, department store or discount store are generally substandard. Find a reputable health food store or stick with a trusted practitioner.

The supplement industry is a $40 billion dollar industry. The required labeling is often fuzzy. Not all Vitamin D, or any other vitamin, have the some efficacy or value. Consumers are often hoodwinked into the latest FAD and buy expensive supplements that may even be filled with adjuvants, fillers, and binders that can be toxic and risky.

Know your source. Read the labels. Get informed. Our patients don't mind paying a little extra when they understand the source of our products and the trust we have been able to place in them.

- B12 – Proper development of villi – sublingual is preferred
- B Complex – supports nervous system and energy
- Vitamin C – prefer Liposomal
- Magnesium – A must for most people (Different forms: Understand there are different forms.)

1esium citrate – constipation, muscle spasms
1esium malate – Fibromyalgia
1esium Glycinate – Better absorption (Also comes in
d for higher dosing.)

Test for magnesium levels by measuring the red blood cell magnesium, also called erythrocyte magnesium (Labcorp or Quest). Most doctors measure it in the serum, which shows how much magnesium is traveling around in the blood.

- Zinc Picolinate – Required for T4-T3 conversion. Best taken with Vitamin C and with food. 25–50 mg
- Omega 3 or Cod Liver Oil – Reduces inflammation

Enzymes

No matter what we eat it all boils down to proteins, carbohydrates and fats. The body then needs to convert these into biochemical substances the body can use. This requires three groups of enzymes:

- Proteolytic – breaks down protein
- Lipolytic – breaks down fat
- Amylolytic – Breaks down Carbohydrates

This process begins long before it reaches the stomach. It begins at first bite (digestive enzymes). The stomach produces between one and two liters of gastric juice each day containing primarily hydrochloric acid and several protein-degrading enzymes such as pepsin and cathepsin.

This hydrochloric acid also destroys some of the bacteria present in the food and promotes the uptake of minerals and trace elements into the bloodstream.

Studies have found that people with Hashimoto's have low stomach acid. This makes it more difficult to digest our proteins and contributes to the fatigue many of us experience. It also leaves food putrefying in the gut and becomes a source of food for the opportunistic bacteria. Low stomach acid can result from a nutrient deficiency, such as thiamin or B12. A good bio-marker on a CBC is to look for the Alkaline Phosphatase. We like to see it at a minimum of 60.

Proteolytic enzymes or systemic enzymes act as immune modulators. This is essential for people with autoimmune disease who can use systemic enzymes to down-regulate the immune response. Systemic enzymes help to break down excess mucus and fibrin. They can replace NSAIDs' for helping with inflammation and provide immune support. Research has shown a reduction in thyroid antibodies when on a systemic enzyme protocol. Can be very helpful in reducing antibodies and regenerating thyroid tissue.

Most of them contain a mix of:

- Bromelain (from pineapple)
- Papain (from papaya)
- Rutin (bioflavonoid)
- Chymotrypsin (porcine)
- Pancreatin (porcine)

A study done with a popular enzyme known as Wobenzym showed that forty people with Hashimoto's were given Systemic Enzymes for 3–6 months and reported a reduction of thyroid symptoms and a decrease in TPO and TG antibodies.

It's important to take them away from food and the best results were seen when taken higher doses than typically recommended. Five capsules three times a day is a good rule of thumb.

Recommended Brands: Wobenzym and Pure Encapsulations

Saccharomyces Boulardii

Saccharomyces Boulardii – is a probiotic that is a yeast instead of a bacteria. This yeast functions like a probiotic in the body. It helps to regulate the intestines and protect them from pathogens, and modulates your immune system by maintaining the integrity of the gut lining.

Ghee

The word "ghee" comes from Sanskrit. Ghee is a form of clarified butter that is a backbone of Ayurveda for health and healing due to its flavor, rich nutritional profile and medicinal value. It is used as a vital food for good digestion, healthy skin, mental clarity and stimulates the secretion of stomach acids to aid in digestion. It is a great alternative for those who are dairy sensitive as the lactose and casein are at trace levels.

It is abundant in butyric acid. Loaded with short chain fatty acids which help to restore the integrity of the gut lining, reduce inflammation and has anti-viral properties.

It's also easy to make at home from unsalted pastured butter.

Recommendation:

Gut Ghee™ is a superior product for gut healing. The ghee is infused with a proprietory blend of essential oil, herbs and spices. formulated by the author for 5 gut types including Toxic, Immune,Candida, Stressed & Gastic gut types.

www.rasahealth.com

Colostrum

Colostrum is the first pre-milk substance that is produced by the mammary gland of female mammals and humans. It is loaded with immune factors and protective proteins. Practitioners are hesitant to recommend it because of the instability of many of the products on the market. Many colostrum supplements are either pasteurized with such high heat that only immunoglobulins remain intact, or are unpasteurized and the pathogens remain. In order for colostrum to be effective, it must contain high levels of the active components, and it must be able to reach the cells with no compromise in bioactivity. We recommend Sovereign Laboratories. Recommended dosages are available on their website. www.sovereignlaboratories.com

Selenium – Reduce TPO antibodies, helps convert T4 – T3. 200–400 mcg on an empty stomach with Vitamin E.

Thiamine or Benfotiamine – Support adrenals, metabolism, and energy – 600 mg per day

Biofilm reduction – An accumulation of microorganisms embedded in a polysaccharide matrix. Biofilm increases the opportunity for gene transfer between bacteria, promoting the spread of bacterial resistance. It prevents normal flora from thriving, minimizes absorption of nutrients.

Curcumin – Anti Inflammatory (if you have a sensitivity to nightshades this may not be right for you).

Dosage – up to 8 grams/day

N-Acetylcysteine (NAC) – A precursor to glutathione. Helps with healing leaky gut and has been found to help reduce thyroid antibodies. 1,800 mg per day with food.

Minerals and Electrolytes – Nearly everyone is deficient. We prefer liquid form for better assimilation.

Apple Cider vinegar

Replace stomach acid. 1 tsp diluted with 2–4 ounces water. Gradually increase to 3–4 tsp.

Recommendation: Bragg's Apple Cider Vinegar

Bone Broth

One of my "go to" favorites. Again, if you ask 10 people for a recipe you will get 10 different recipes, and that is because bone broth is as ancient as time. Early tribes understood the nourishment and healing powers of bones and oral traditions carried these recipes forward.

Having made hundreds of different combinations, I am still learning. I tell my patients, "Just start. Pick a recipe that appeals to you and just get started." The benefits way outnumber any inconvenience, so let me tell you about some of them.

Amino Acids – Amino acids are the building blocks of protein. Think of a Lego set. If you are missing 3 of 6 pieces needed to build a rocket ship, you may end up with an airplane at best. Same thing with amino acids. We need ALL of them, and that is what bone broth provides. Proline and glycine are two amino acids that work together to build collagen and cartilage. Glycine aids with digestion by improving gastric acid secretion and is a precursor for glutathione – a very important antioxidant.

Glutamine is critical to gut health and aids detoxification – is also abundant in bone broth. Millions of Americans suffer from joint pain and are found to be low in amino acids. Proline and glycine are particularly helpful for our joints.

We have two different types of cartilage – fibrous and hyaline. One is dense and the other is thin. Made up largely of type 2 collagen, cartilage can be worn down over time. Whether you have knee pain, tendon damage, bone density issues, or wear and tear, drinking bone broth daily will help rebuild and replenish the nutrients necessary.

Collagen turns into gelatin (the jiggly layer) found across the top of cooled bone broth. I remember my mother drinking Knox gelatin in the 60's, as it helped to repair nails, hair, and skin.

Marrow: Did you know when hunting prey, animals will first consume the marrow? This is due to its nutrient density. It is an abundant source of natural gelatin and Vitamin A. If you were to do an evolutionary history of nutrition, bone marrow would be a great case study.

Grass fed and organic do matter. I have tried making broth from conventional stores, and what I have noticed as the biggest difference is how the broth smells. When you are simmering broth for 24 or more hours, the odor wafts throughout the house all night long. We have noticed that the odor from non-grass fed, non-free range bones is exceptionally harsh. It may be that the toxic buildup in the bones is significantly higher and this is being released as well.

I have also found that roasting the bones in the oven at 350 degrees for 30 minutes helps builds a savory broth, and I typically mix a variety of bones together, using everything from chicken feet, necks, and backs to knuckles, feet, and legs.

Recommendation:

Westonpricefoundation.org has a wealth of information on where to find the resources you need. Sally Fallon wrote *Nourished Traditions,* and I recommend it to every patient for finding the recipe that is right for them.

Gut Butter – Chronic GI Support

½ C of Extra Virgin Olive Oil
½ lb Raw organic grass-fed butter
8 Caps Therbiotic Complete
8 Caps Colostrum (or 5,000 mg of powder)
L-Glutamine 3,000 mg
Zn-carnosine 150 mg
Butyric Cal Mag by Biotics (4 capsules)
2 Tbsp raw honey
Sialex 400 mg – Ecological formulas

Mix ingredients, then refrigerate

Dosing: 2 Tbsp /day for 2 weeks
Then 1 Tsp per day for 2 weeks
Then 1 Tbsp per day for 1 month

Can be put on food or eaten plain. Let melt in mouth if possible.

Gas and bloating

- Slowly increase fiber
- Eliminate dairy
- Soak beans and grains before cooking

- Find the trigger
- Use digestive bitters
- Functional testing
- IgG food sensitivity testing
- Comprehensive Stool Analysis (CSA) for Candida and parasites
- Small Intestinal Bacterial Overgrowth (SIBO) hydrogen breath test
- Chew your food well
- Colon massage
- Constipation

Eat and poop

This is the ideal progression. It's interesting to me when we ask patients about their bowel movements and they respond, "they're normal." Normal is eat and poop with a transit time of between 12–24 hours. Transit time is the length it takes for food to travel through the digestive tract. Isn't this what babies do?

If you are only moving your bowels once per day or less than, then you are constipated. Persistent constipation is a red flag.

- Lifestyle Treatment
- Increase exercise
- Evaluate medications that may be constipating
- Consume more fiber
- Stay hydrated
- Eliminate dairy
- Soak dried figs or prunes overnight; drink the water
- Vitamin C, magnesium, aloe vera juice, slippery elm, psyllium, marshmallow root
- Essential oils of rosemary, fennel

Diarrhea

- Saccharomyces boulardii
- L-glutamine

- Aloe Vera juice
- Reduce triggers
- Bentonite Clay
- Zinc
- Deglycyrrhizinated licorice (DG)
- BRAT diet: banana, rice, apples, toast
- Broths
- Eat for your Microbiome

Learn to test

Practitioner recommendation:

Autonomic Response Testing

http://rasahealth.com/what-is-autonomic-response-testing/

http://www.klinghardtacademy.com/

Consumer:

This on-line course has received high acclaim

http://www.epiphanyhealingarts.com/muscle-testing-made-easy.html

www.klinghardtacademy.com – certified practitioners

Chiropractic Adjustment

Long before I became a doctor of chiropractic I benefited from seeing a chiropractor. In fact, I saw it as "early prevention – not early detection." In those days I did not have the science or knowledge to understand the vitalistic model of chiropractic – I only know that I always "felt" better...my runny nose would stop – my sinuses cleared up – my mood got better and my strength and energy returned.

Chiropractors recognize the body is a self-healing, self-generating organism and given no interference will function at optimal levels. Chiropractors understand the connection between the body, mind and spirit and are taught that the Autonomic Nervous System is the controller of all function in the body on the physical/energetic level. The ANS impacts how we digest, eliminate, metabolize, sleep and many other functions. It simply makes sense to me to keep your ANS healthy and subluxation free.

A chiropractic adjustment does not treat thyroid disease but it does help the person who has thyroid dis-ease. A chiropractor skilled in Applied Kinesiology will evaluate the teres minor muscle which is associated with the thyroid. A high percentage of patients will have a standing posture of one or both arms internally rotated so that the palms face more posteriorly because of weakness of the teres minor muscle.

One of the "adjustments" your chiropractor may make is to evaluate and treat the Ileocecal valve. (ICV) The primary function of the ICV is to control the flow of food from the small intestine to the large intestine. The small intestine is where most of the nutrients are absorbed and large intestine is where the waste is processed before excretion.

The main functions of the ICV are to:

1. Make sure that waste doesn't stay too long in the small intestine.
2. To prevent back-flow from the large intestine to the small intestine, this stops bacteria-laden waste from comtaminating the small intestine a major problem in SIBO (small intestine bacterial overgrowth)

The ICV functions primarily under the control of the nervous system and the vagus nerve. It is generally accepted that it is open by sympathetic and closed by parasympathetic action.Because of various contributing factors, the ICV can sometimes malfunction. As this happens, toxic waste is able to re-enter the small intestine where it is absorbed, causing the spread of toxins throughout the body and thus stressing the liver and the immune system, which then has to work hard to eliminate the toxins and their effects. Toxins that cannot be eliminated are stored in the body in the joints

The main causes if ICV malfunction are:

- Caffeine
- Low stomach acid
- refined sugars and sweeteners
- Chocolate
- Tobacco
- Alcohol
- Antibiotics
- Stress
- Lack of sleep
- Poor posture
- Lack of exercise
- Dehydration
- Pathogenic bacteria
- Viruses
- Candida

Symptoms of a closed or open ICV:

- Palpitations
- Headaches
- Migraines
- Pseudo-Meniere's syndrome
- Right shoulder pain
- Nausea
- Faintness
- Fluid retention
- Tinnitus
- Pseudo sinus infection
- Sudden thirst
- Dark circles under the eyes
- Fatigue
- Right leg weakness
- General aches and pains

Therapeutic Pure Essential Oils

Essential oils have been a part of my personal and professional life for 25 years. I've always been drawn to the power of scent and and have studied the physiological shifts that are impacted when we smell. This knowledge is so common that this is why many major food stores will greet you with the smell of cinnamon and vanilla. They understand the body interprets this via a chemical messenger that lights up a part of our brain where we store memory. Realtors stage open houses with apples or cookies in the oven because when we experience those smells it invites feelings of nesting, home, and gathering.

Smell is only one way of experiencing the oils. You can simply place a drop in your hand and rub your hands together and bring them to your nose and inhale, or you can use a diffuser and fill a room with your favorite healing and therapeutic essential oil. Certain oils can be taken internally. We often dilute them in a gelatin capsule you can purchase at a health food store and mix the essential oil with fractionated coconut oil. Some oils can be added to water, and you can gargle with them or swallow directly. Taking them internally versus placing them topically offers different benefits. When in doubt, just smell it. You can safely place oils on the bottom of the feet, either diluted or neat. Either way, the therapeutic effects will be absorbed and delivered into the bloodstream.

We have reflex points on the soles of our feet and our ears that refer to the gut, thyroid, and adrenals. You can find these charts online and use them as a guide as to where to place the oils.

Think of essential oils as a spice cabinet for the body. Just as you learned the flavors of thyme, oregano, and pepper for cooking, and how and when to use them, you will also learn over time the best oil to use at the best time for the best reason.

One of the challenges when sharing the therapeutic benefits of essential oils is that no two peppermint or lemon or any other essential oils carry the same healing benefits. Soil, location, quality, and harvesting all have an impact on the therapeutic value. I have worked with two different companies and I am sure there are others, but I have experienced the value of oils from Young Living and DoTerra. Quality does matter. Not all peppermint and lavender is created equal. Frankincense is one of my "go to" oils, and the constituents of frankincense will change depending on where the oil was harvested, who harvested it, and by what means. If you do a pubmed search on Frankincense Boswellia, you will find studies showing its usefulness in everything from inflammation to cancer and viruses to pain. In my opinion, this oil belongs in everyone's medicine cabinet.

Essential oils contain a variety of compounds with names like monoterpenes, sesquiterpenes, and aldehydes. Each of these compounds are known for different effects.

Monoterpenes are known to be antibacterial, antiviral, and act as a decongestant. Aldehydes are anti-inflammatory, sedating, calming. Oils with aldehydes are Lemongrass, Lavender, Roman Chamomile, and Melissa. Sesquiterpenes are also anti-inflammatory, immune stimulating, and increase bile flow from the liver. This can be helpful in an autoimmune condition. Myrrh, Melissa, Basic, and German Chamomile can be helpful here.

Remember earlier we talked about "quorum sensing," the communication that the microbiome uses? When we are healing the gut it is important to break down the biofilm and inhibit this quorum sensing. Oregano is one of the essential oils that has shown the ability to do this.

Thyme oil contains a compound that has been shown to interact with surface proteins of bacteria, leading to an alteration of the cell surface and interrupting the initial attachment phase of biofilm formation.

Oil recommendations for Healing Hashimoto's and Healing the Gut

Thyroid Support – Combine the following:

25 drops Lemongrass – Thyroid, digestive, emotional balance
25 drops Clove – emotional balance, thyroid & metabolism, immune boost
10 drops Frankincense – Immune system, depression, emotional balance, trauma

4 drops Peppermint – Excellent for headaches, hot flashes, anti-inflammatory, invigorating

Prepare the above blend in a 10 ml roller bottle with fractionated coconut oil and apply topically to thyroid and reflexology points 3x daily.

Essential Oils for the Gut

- Stomach – Black pepper, fennel, ginger, wild orange
- Intestinal lining – grapefruit, peppermint
- Good night's sleep – Serenity, Lavender, Cedarwood, and Vetiver
- Adrenal support – Basil and Rosemary
- Digestive system support – DigestZen, Ginger, Lemongrass, and Fennel

Can apply oils to abdomen, use a warm compress, or place a drop into the naval.

Increasing Parasympathetic response – It is this part of the autonomic nervous system that helps with repair and replenishment. Use this blend as de-stressor and to lessen anxiety.

5 drops Rose essential oil
10 drops patchouli
20 drops lavender
20 drops wild orange

Prepare the above blend in a 10ml roller bottle with fractionated coconut oil and apply topically to thyroid and reflexology points 3x daily

There are also therapies like Aroma Touch and Raindrop, which can be stand-alone treatments. These are layering of essential oils applied along the spine for deep relaxation, absorption, and therapeutic healing for inflammation, pain, trauma, emotional and immune enhancing.

Consider unhealed emotional wounds

Every physical condition has an underlying emotional component.

Our practice embraces a philosophy called the "5 Levels of Health & Healing" as taught by Dr. Klinghardt.

The 5 levels of health and healing include the physical body, energy body, mental body, informational, and consciousness. This model helps us identify underlying emotional wounds that may be conscious or unconscious.

One of the tools we have available in our office helps us to identify what this emotional wound may be for any given patient. Sometimes these feelings are unconscious.

When stomach/gut issues light up for a patient, we often find the underlying cause as being:

A past conflict or confrontation which leads to a situation that cannot be accepted or digested. it may be in connection with fear of starvation in the broadest sense, e.g., loss of job or business and not being able to afford food. It may involve something that was said or seen that could not be taken in... Instead it sits in the belly, festering, living with indigestible anger and denial of facts.

Using the same tool, when the thyroid or throat area is highlighted it will indicate issues around "not being able to speak for fear of rejection, misunderstanding, confrontation, etc., and/or not being able to find one's voice."

Louise Hay wrote in *Heal Your Body:*

Thyroid issues may have their roots in a feeling of humiliation. I never get to do what I want to do and/or when is it going to be my turn? Hay suggests this affirmation: *"I move beyond old limitations and now allow myself to express freely and creatively."*

What is very interesting about this concept is we find that this type of unresolved emotions and emotional stress impacts our bodies in multiple ways. The digestive and immune systems can become compromised, resulting in lowered hydrochloric acid and increased cortisol.

The beauty of pure essential oils is that they carry energetic signatures that have been shown to be beneficial to healing emotions and chronic stress, working beyond the chemistry of our physical bodies, but opening the door to our unconscious and deep emotional space. When you find one product that works on more than one of the five levels of healing, it instantly becomes a valued source of healing.

Essential oils & Emotions

Some therapies we use and or recommend for our patients:

Applied Psychoneurobiology
Emotional Freedom Technique and all the offshoots
Neuro-Emotional Technique (NET)

Addressing the emotional factor will ALWAYS move the patient into a greater state of homeostasis. It is sometimes the last place patients look for answers and is often where they receive the greatest benefit.

Recommended oils for emotional cleansing and clearing:

Lavender

The Oil of Communication. We talked about the thyroid being related to issues with finding one's voice. Our voice box is located in the neck which is the area of our 5th Chakra. The 5th chakra when balanced inspires speech, it is the center for communicating our truth to the world. It is about giving voice to our inner heart and is represented by the color blue.

Lavender applied to this area or inhaled can begin to assist in resolving any blockages around being "seen and heard." Lavender supports us in releasing the tension and constriction that may stem from fear of expressing one's self.

Frankincense

The Oil of Truth. Frankincense helps us to remember and reconnect with our spiritual understanding, gifts, wisdom, and knowledge the soul brought into the world.

Especially helpful for anyone that may have felt abandoned and/or forgotten or unprotected.

Clove

The Oil of Boundaries. We often see in issues around "boundaries" in gut problems. Clove helps us to find appropriate boundaries and defenses. This oil is especially helpful in anyone who may have felt defeated, intimidated, or dominated.

For help with "energetic" boundaries we turn to Melaleuca.

White Fir

The Oil of Generational Healing. We talked about Hashimoto's needing three components: genetic, impaired gut, and toxins and/or infection. White Fir helps us break generational and destructive patterns such as addiction, anger, and eating disorders.

Tension Blend

The Oil of Relief. This is a blend of wintergreen, lavender, peppermint, frankincense, cilantro, roman chamomile, and marjoram (available through DoTerra).

It helps us to release stress and emotional tension, and release fears that create pain in the physical body. Tension Blend can help soothe trauma and bring balance to the body and energy body.

I find it interesting that the thyroid gland is shaped like a butterfly. When we think about the stages of a butterfly's life, we know there are transitions and transformation. This is also true when healing the thyroid from an emotional level. Be willing to get still and look within. Ask to be shown what may be standing between you and complete healing. What is revealed to you and what is asking to be healed?

Chapter Summary

- ✓ Real food does not come in a box
- ✓ Learn to test
- ✓ What is good today may not be good tomorrow
- ✓ Eat to heal your microbiome
- ✓ Consider unhealed trauma
- ✓ Address undigested issues
- ✓ Use tools to address the stress
- ✓ The solution is different for each of us

Gut Bless You

As I've been writing *Heal Hashimoto's: Start with the Gut,* the world is still going on outside my window. We are in a political season unlike any other as we observe well-intentioned presidential candidates debate their positions. One candidate believes we need to "win" and "build walls." Another candidate feels differently. They say we need to make America "whole" again and build bridges.

In the evolving world of science, a major breakthrough has been established that Einstein was correct when he hypothesized that time and space were each simply extensions of the other, and microbiome medicine is now focusing more on the bacteria and their genes than the germs and human genome.

What do they have in common? They each are asking us to look beyond our current understanding of what we perceive of how things work. They each are suggesting that there is a unified field or force that governs the whole, and the best solutions are those that unify and bring about the greatest good for all.

As you learn about the microbiome, you will see that they use "quorum sensing" to communicate as they evolve and move together for the common good of all, even if that means having to sacrifice one for the many. They seem to have an intuitive sense that what is good for the whole is best for the one, and ask their individual parts to make choices based on the greatest good for all. They know how to adapt and reinvent themselves depending on the environmental conditions they are exposed to by their host. They have a common goal and that is to thrive.

What does this have to do with the gut?

It turns out this "social network" that outnumbers human cells ten to one is the very foundation of health. We used to think microbes in the body were pathogenic, and researchers focused solely on these harmful bugs and ignored the possible importance of the rest. It turns out that our microbiome is as unique as your fingerprint. No two people share the same microbial makeup – even identical twins. What's more, the commensal bacteria play a major role in both digestion and the regulation of appetite.

Bacteroides thetaiotaomicron is a champion carbohydrate chomper, capable of breaking down the large, complex carbohydrates found in many plant foods into glucose and digestible sugars, and while the human genome lacks most of the genes required to make the enzymes that degrade these complex carbohydrates, Bacteroides have genes that code for more than 260 enzymes capable of digesting plant matter. Think of the microbiome as "friends with benefits." This delicate balance of commensal, mutualistic, and pathogenic microbiota are the drivers of assimilation, absorption, and excretion. As an acquired and essential organ of the body, the gut microbiota provide a wide variety of beneficial functions, including: gleaning indigestible ingredients from food and synthesizing nutritional factors such as vitamins; detoxifying harmful chemicals from the environment; they help us develop a robust systemic and intestinal immune system; provide signals for epithelial renewal to maintain gut integrity; and secrete anti-microbial products, which select against pathogenic bacteria through the development of colonization resistance.

And they work together as a whole. Just as space-time is a continuum, so is the microbiome and YOU! Every thought, action, and food has an impact on how these microbiota behave. Bacteroides fragilis help to keep the immune system in balance by boosting its anti-inflammatory arm. When researchers injected mice with B. Fragilis, the balance between the pro-inflammatory and anti-inflammatory T-cells was restored.

Because of the lifestyle changes over the past century, the widespread use of antibiotics, changes in human ecology, and the dramatic increase in the number of deliveries by Caesarean section have taken a toll on the human microbiome, reducing the variety of bacteria to which we are exposed. Organisms like B. fragilis are disappearing. We have completely changed our association with the microbial world. One microbiologist, Masmanian, says, "In our efforts to distance ourselves from disease-causing infectious agents, we have probably also changed our associations with beneficial organisms. Our intentions are good, but there's a price to pay."

In the case of B. fragilis, the price may be a significant increase in the number of autoimmune disorders. Masmanian contends that the recent sevenfold to eightfold increase in rates of autoimmune disorders is related to the decline in beneficial microbes.

Our medical leaders have told us to "fear" the sun for the damage it may do and we have stopped venturing out for a beautiful sunrise or sunset.

Instead of opening the windows for "fresh" air, we now have been told to believe it comes in an aerosol spray can, and if we want the whitest and cleanest laundry we need to add chemicals and softeners instead of hanging them out on a clothesline.

Food stores contain very little real food. In fact, if you want "living foods" you will be limited to the outside periphery of the store. The other 13 isles will be filled with boxed, processed, chemically-treated ingredients that we have come to call "food."

Caesarean birth has nearly replaced vaginal birth, where we have the first chance to receive a healthy inoculation of microbiota from our moms. Remember my conversation with the the OB-Gyn friend who told me doctors are paid the same whether it's a vaginal birth or C-section, but the big difference is in the liability? A doctor is more likely to be protected if something goes wrong and they chose a C-section than if they had gone with a vaginal birth. Makes one wonder how the very act of nature, giving birth, has now been relegated to an operational suite. Interesting fact, doctors are paid the very same with both procedures. So who is making the extra dollars? Hospitals and insurance companies.

This scenario plays out with thyroid health as well. Conventional wisdom for diagnosing thyroid disorders is based on outdated and somewhat flawed science. When scientists first set the "normal" ranges of TSH for healthy individuals, they also included the elderly and those with a compromised thyroid function, leading to calculations that skewed the findings. This resulted in patients who fell outside this range being told their tests were "normal."

Not only that, but they are relying on a test that is often misleading as levels of circulating hormones may be different at different times.

According to Izabella Wentz, author of *Hashimoto's Thyroiditis: Finding the Root Cause* it is only in recent years, The National Academy of Clinical Biochemists indicated that 95% of individuals without thyroid disease have TSH concentrations below 2.5 µIU/L, and a new normal reference range was defined by the American College of Clinical Endocrinologists to be between 0.3- 3.0 µIU/ml. Functional medicine practitioners have further defined that the normal reference range should be under 2

However, most labs have not adjusted that range in the reports they provide to physicians, and have kept ranges as lax as 0.2–8.0 µIU/ml. Most physicians only look for values outside of the "normal" reference range provided by the labs, and may not be familiar with the new guidelines. Thus, many physicians may miss the patients who are showing an elevated TSH.

Then came Synthroid. In 2013 and 2014, Synthroid was the #1 prescribed drug in all of the United States (based on number of prescriptions filled). This is a synthetic version of one of our active thyroid hormones, levothyroxine (T4). This medication works wonders for many people with Hashimoto's and hypothyroidism, but some continue to struggle with hypothyroid symptoms, even when taking the correct dose of T4.

This is because T4 is a precursor hormone, and it needs to be activated to T3 (liothyronine), to be available to the body. Many people do not convert T4 to T3 adequately. In those cases, thyroid patients find that adding T3 directly to their bodies can make a big difference in how they feel.

Patients often report their doctor will not prescribe anything but Synthroid. So what makes endocrinologists so skeptical? Doctors are required to follow guidelines according to the "standard of care." T4 Levothyroxine is most often cited in studies, whereas Armour, Nature-Throid, and WP are derived from the thyroid glands of animals and were more difficult to assay. The lab with the deeper pockets and stronger sales force makes a big impact over smaller labs. Even when studies were published to show the alternatives were equivalent and cheaper for patients, the damage had been done and many doctors were unwilling and/or lacked the knowledge to consider all the options. Clinical trials are very expensive and require funding.

Find a practitioner that considers the whole picture and relies on more than the TSH.

As the world revolves outside my window, science is reporting new findings of gravitational waves. In the early 1900's Einstein was ridiculed for his hypothesis that time and space are a unified continuum or "fabric." He predicted that the acceleration of massive objects would churn the fabric of the space-time continuum, which would cause waves to form, much like the waves that emerge in water when you throw a pebble into a pond.

This has recently been confirmed. It means that time is flexible – it's not the constant thing we imagine it to be. Time will flow differently for people under differing conditions. Even issues like the sequence of events can be different for people traveling in separate directions at significant speed. Can you conceive of time and space actually being just one thing, bending and flowing in response to other forces? This suggests that each of us, with every thought, word, and deed, has an impact on the whole. How we move together – or not – ultimately will decide the outcome.

The Garden of Eden is in the Gut.

Having been raised by a Catholic father and a Presbyterian mom, I had early roots in Sunday school and Bible studies. Even an atheist can find the story of the Garden of Eden a metaphorical wonder.

"The Lord God took the man and put him in the Garden of Eden to work it and take care of it. 1:6 And the Lord God commanded the man, "You are free to eat from any tree in the garden."

Now the serpent was more crafty than any of the wild animals the Lord God had made. He said to the woman, "Did God really say, 'You must not eat from any tree in the garden'?"

2 The woman said to the serpent, "We may eat fruit from the trees in the garden, 3 but God did say, 'You must not eat fruit from the tree that is in the middle of the garden, and you must not touch it, or you will die.'"

From a metaphorical perspective, is the Garden of Eden really the rich and diverse health-giving microbiota that are the foundation to life? Is the serpent the additives, processed foods, sugar, and chemicals that initiate changes in our behavior that make us crave the very things that hurt us? Was Jesus telling us to look to the Tree? Our sustenance comes when we harvest our food from the vines and soil and bushes. Is the Garden of Eden where the microbiome have evolved over billions of years? Is it possible that the story in Genesis was the earliest reference to the Garden in our Gut?

Just as you would nurture a garden with water, sunlight, and bacteria, so too shall we find health when we nourish ourselves with the same. If you want health, seek it from within.

Diversity is the secret to a healthy gut. Diversity is the secret to humanity.

Diversity and harmony.

Gut Bless you!

Resources

Certified Hashimoto's Practitioners

www.hashimotoinstitute.com

Certified Autonomic Response Testing Practitioners

www.klinghardtacademy.com

Applied Kinesiology

http://www.icakusa.com/

Functional Medicine

www.myfunctionalmedicinedoctor.org

Fermented Foods

www.wildbrine.com

www.wisechoicemarket.com

www.baofoodanddrink.com

Grass-Fed Pasture Raised Bones

http://www.westonaprice.org/

Market Supplies

Thrive Market

www.thrivemarket.com

US Wellness Meats

www.grasslandbeef.com

Vital Choice Wild Seafood and Organics

www.vitalchoice.com

Certified pure therapeutic grade essential oils

www.mydoterra.com/rasahealth

Supplements for Support

Dispensed by Health Professionals Only

Physica Energetics

www.thorne.com

www.metagenics.com

Emotional Support/Energy Medicine

http://askandreceive.org/

www.netmindbody.com

Thyroid Guide

http://getrealthyroid.com/the-real-resources/my-thyroid-guide/

Lab Testing

www.23andme.com

www.gdx.net

www.ubiome.com

www.biohealth.com

Dr. Rasa Community and support

www.rasahealth.com

Facebook: https://www.facebook.com/raSahealth/

Facebook: Essential Oils community
https://www.facebook.com/doterra.drrasa/

GMO Shopping guide

http://nongmoshoppingguide.com/

About the Author

Dr. Sharon Lee Rasa is a doctor of natural medicine and a pioneer in holistic health. She is a doctor of chiropractic, functional medicine and a leader at the cutting edge of the new frontier in understanding health from a multi-level model. After her mother was sent home at the age of 51 with a "we've done all we can" prognosis, Dr. Rasa's life path set sail in a new direction at the age of 25: to understand health and healing from a holistic and integrative perspective. Dr. Rasa has three decades of studies, research, practicing, teaching, and writing in the field of holistic and functional medicine.

She embraces the body as a self-healing, self-organizing, self-regulating organism when given no interference.

Having suffered from Lyme Disease, mold toxicity, and Hashimoto's, Dr. Rasa embraced her own healing in an effort to not only help herself but thousands of others. She has a private practice in Red Bank, NJ.

In parting, we have a gift for you. Get instant access to Dr. Rasa's e-book "How to Create a Healthy Kitchen" and we will keep you informed of upcoming webinars, events and trainings.

http://rasahealth.com/health-kitchen-gift/

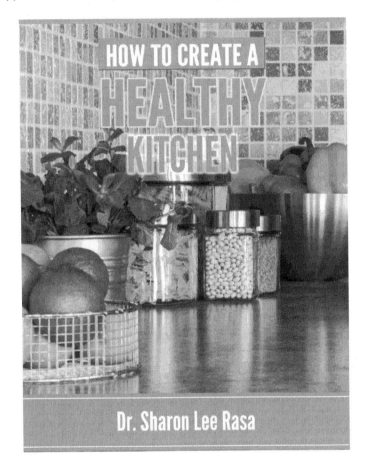

Would you kindly take a moment?

Thank you for buying my book! Thousands of people are in need of information to help them navigate the slippery slope of Hashimoto's. Your comments will help to make it easier for the next person who may find him or herself there. I really appreciate all of your feedback, and I love hearing what you have to say. It is your input that will make the next version better.

Please leave us a helpful REVIEW on Amazon.

Made in the USA
San Bernardino, CA
06 November 2016